1/1988　　　£22-50

R.O.H School of Physiotherapy
Students' Library

Lending Section

TREATMENT WITH INTERFERENTIAL CURRENT

TREATMENT WITH INTERFERENTIAL CURRENT

LILYANA NIKOLOVA MD DSc

Professor of Physiotherapy and Rehabilitation,
Chair of Physiotherapy and Rehabilitation,
The Medical Academy, Sofia, Bulgaria

Foreword by
Jeanne-Marie Ganne MCSP DipTP MAPA FACP
President of the Australian College of Physiotherapists;
formerly Senior Lecturer in Physiotherapy, South
Australian Institute of Technology, Adelaide

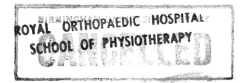

Churchill Livingstone

EDINBURGH LONDON MELBOURNE AND NEW YORK 1987

CHURCHILL LIVINGSTONE
Medical Division of Longman Group UK Limited

Distributed in the United States of America by Churchill
Livingstone Inc., 1560 Broadway, New York, N.Y. 10036,
and by associated companies, branches and representatives
throughout the world.

First and second editions published in Bulgarian
© Lilyana Nikolova c/o JUSAUTOR, Sofia, 1971, 1979
First edition in English based on the second Bulgarian
edition, revised and expanded
© Longman Group UK Limited 1987

ISBN 0-443-03172-X

British Library Cataloguing in Publication Data
Nikolova, Lilyana
   Treatment with interferential current.
   1. Electrotherapeutics
   I. Title
   615.8'45   RM871

Library of Congress Cataloging in Publication Data
Nikolova, Lilyana.
   Treatment with interferential current.
   "First edition in English based on the second Bulgarian edition, revised and
expanded" — T.p. verso.
   Bibliography: p.
   Includes index.
   1. Electrotherapeutics.   I. Nikolova, Lilyana.
Lechenie s interferenten tok.   II. Title.
[DNLM: 1. Electrotherapy. WB 495 N6928t]
RM871.N69 1986   615.8'45   86–17592

1782323

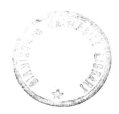

Produced by Longman Singapore Publishers Pte Ltd
Printed in Singapore

Foreword

It is a pleasure to have the opportunity of acknowledging Professor Nikolova's major contribution to interferential therapy.

English-speaking physiotherapists will welcome this book, which is a record of the author's vast clinical experience of the use of interference currents over a period of 23 years.

Twenty years ago, few physiotherapists had heard of interferential therapy in Great Britain and Australia, and very few had used it clinically. There was at the time in the United Kingdom a phase of diminishing interest in the therapeutic use of direct and low frequency electrical currents, apart from faradic or faradic equivalent currents to produce motor stimulation. In the United States interferential therapy was virtually unknown. Although the original work of Dr H. Nemec was followed up on the European continent, and early reports of treatment and clinical investigations were presented at conferences and published in European journals, it was difficult to obtain information on the subject in the English language.

Professor Nikolova became a generous source of information to any physiotherapist who sought her assistance from abroad. Her early recognition of the advantages and potential value of interferential therapy and her extensive experience of its use for a wide variety of inflammatory and traumatic conditions have effectively contributed to its development in many treatment centres.

Interferential therapy was introduced in physiotherapy teaching units and clinical departments in Adelaide in 1971. Professor Nikolova's work on fractures also stimulated the introduction of this treatment for delayed union in Adelaide in 1974. She was an early pioneer in drawing attention to the effects of these currents in hastening resolution of inflammation and tissue regeneration, in addition to their analgesic effect. This prompted her early use of interference currents in the treatment of fracture complications and to promote repair of bone, showing the advantages of a non-invasive technique which stimulates both soft tissues and bone. This was in contrast to the numerous experiments carried out by various research workers which led, in the 1970s, to surgical implantation of electrodes at fracture sites in order to stimulate callus formation with small amounts of direct or pulsed currents, given continuously.

Professor Nikolova's clinical observations of the results of treatment prompted her to undertake the experimental studies detailed in the second chapter of this book. Results of these histochemical studies showing the effects of interferential therapy on capillaries and on the activity of certain enzymes should be of special interest to those who have presumed that metabolic changes must occur at cellular levels.

The author does not set out to present the complex physics of these currents, and she also recognises that the effects of different frequencies require further investigation. The major value of this book is in the reports of clinical treatment, in the physiological tests used to determine results objectively and in some comparisons of the effects of various treatments. As a Professor of Physiotherapy and Rehabilitation, Doctor of Science and medical practitioner, the author points out the importance of a combined approach in treatment, where indicated, and how interferential therapy can supplement or be supplemented by additional therapy, including chemotherapy.

Whereas there has been a tendency to use interferential therapy principally in the treatment of musculo-skeletal problems, the author stresses its value for vascular abnormalities such as Sudeck's atrophy, for pelvic inflammatory disease and sterility, in the treatment of nerve lesions and some visceral chronic conditions. Because of the basic metabolic effects described in the chapter on histochemical research, the effects on pain and sympathetic control, the penetration of the currents, the absence of any unpleasant sensation and few contra-indications, it is to be expected that these currents can have a wide application.

Although the clinical reports frequently refer to treatment of chronic complications and cases whose early management proved inadequate, the author emphasises the importance of early application of the currents which shortens the total number of treatments required and obtains the best results. She recommends that an adequate trial of treatment with interferential therapy should be completed, in many cases, before resorting to surgery.

With renewed interest in the effects and uses of electrical currents and electro-magnetic fields in medicine and in view of the constantly rising costs of health services, it is important for the medical profession to be aware of the value of therapy which can play a part in preventing prolonged disability and the need for very costly procedures. It is equally important for physiotherapists to use these currents with appropriate understanding and careful skill and to evaluate different techniques themselves.

There is no doubt that this book will be a valuable source of clinical information to readers, and I am indebted to the author for her extensive contribution in this area.

Adelaide

Jeanne-Marie Ganne

Preface

Treatment with interferential current plays an important role in the rehabilitation of patients with a number of diseases (for example, fractures of bones and their complications and injuries to peripheral nerves). It not only promotes maximum restoration of function of patients, but also shortens the duration of the healing process (i.e. the treatment time), which is of great importance from both an economic and a social point of view. Unfortunately, in spite of these benefits interferential therapy has not yet found the necessary extensive and timely application in clinical practice.

Interferential therapy in Bulgaria was first applied by myself and my colleagues in 1963. The first edition of our book *Treatment with Interferential Current* (Sofia, 1971) was a summary of the experience gained up to that period from the clinical application of interferential current in the treatment of various diseases. The second edition (Sofia, 1979) was expanded with new chapters and the latest indications for treatment with interferential current for diseases such as exogenous toxic hepatitis and adnexal sterility. This present edition in English has been thoroughly revised and expanded to include experimental and clinical investigations. The experimental studies conducted contribute to the elucidation of the mechanism of action of interferential current and its advantages over other electrotherapeutic methods.

Our book aims to further the wider application of interferential therapy in medical practice in all diseases for which it is suited or for which it can be considered a method of choice. It is intended not only for physiotherapists, but also for clinicians of all specialties.

Sofia, 1987   L.N.

Contents

PART | ONE

Introduction

1

Introduction to interferential therapy

GENERAL DATA ON INTERFERENTIAL CURRENT

Interferential current (IC) was suggested for therapeutic application by the Austrian scientist H. Nemec in 1949. To obtain interferential current, two medium-frequency currents of say 4000 and 4100 Hz are used. These two alternating currents of medium frequency are induced into the underlying tissues separately so that they cross in the treatment field perpendicular to each other (Fig. 1.1a). For that purpose four leads with four electrodes are applied, two for each circuit (Fig. 1.1b).

One of the currents is always introduced at a constant frequency, e.g. 4000 Hz, while the frequency of the second one is variable, e.g. between 4000 and 4100 Hz, the difference between the two currents being from 0 to 100 Hz. At the crossover point of these two completely distinct currents of medium frequency within the tissues, a new, biologically active low-frequency current is produced. The frequency of the new IC thus produced corresponds exactly to the difference between the two component currents, i.e. it varies between 0 and 100 Hz. For instance, if the first current is of a constant frequency of 4000 Hz, and the second one of 4001 Hz, then the resultant frequency is 1 Hz; if the second one has a frequency of 4050 Hz, then the resultant one is 50 Hz. The difference chosen depends on therapeutic requirements. The main new concept is that the effective current is not introduced from outside, but is produced in depth, or endoge-

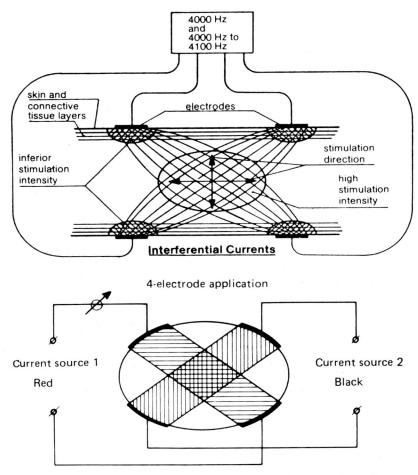

Fig. 1.1 a. Diagram representing generation of interferential current (according to Hansjürgens). b. Leads and electrodes.

nously, within the tissues and organs of the human body. The newly produced endogenous current is of a low frequency. These are two essential advantages from a therapeutic point of view. What is their significance for therapy?

Low-frequency current has a stimulating effect on excitable tissues. The maximum stimulation is close to the surface in the vicinity of the electrodes, diminishing considerably in depth. In order to reach deep-lying organs and tissues, a current of intolerable intensity must be applied. If it is of tolerable intensity, it is ineffective in depth.

Medium-frequency current of a constant intensity, even if the latter is high, does not provoke skin irritation and its application is painless. This makes it possible to provide treatment with a higher intensity of current and thus raise the activity of the generated endogenous interferential current. Its advantage is not only that it is painless, but also that it acts in depth without damage to the underlying tissues. In other words, whereas with other low-frequency currents the highest excitation is under the electrodes and drops when induced in the body, the most important features of IC is its effect on tissues lying between the electrodes.

Various interferential therapy (IT) units have been designed and are constantly being improved. The present book is not aimed at considering the technical data and advantages of the different units (they are demonstrated in suppliers' cata-

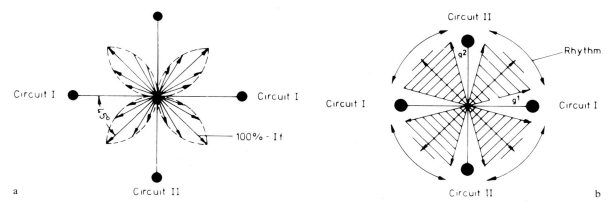

Fig. 1.2 a. Static interferential field. b. Dynamic interferential field.

logues), but to present the results of research work and accumulated clinical experience on the effects of interferential therapy. We should note, however, the significance of the dynamic interferential field. With a square position of the electrodes and a homogenous 'patient environment' the interferential field at the crossover point is uneven, but is distributed according to exact physical laws. A static interferential field is thus produced with a specific distribution of the interferential intensity. The *interference* is zero within connecting lines between the electrodes of the same circuit (Fig. 1.2a). However, the interferential effect rises as one moves away from these points in either direction, the maximum 100% interference being reached at an angle of 45°. In modern units a device is provided to move automatically and rhythmically the static interferential field, thus a dynamic interferential current is produced passing through the whole area subject to treatment[1] (Fig. 1.2b).

Dynamic interferential current is reported to gain better and faster therapeutic results than a static interferential field, but in fact they have a similar healing effect (Hansjürgens, 1974; Nippel, 1979; Laabs et al, 1982a,b; de Domenico, 1981, 1982). Thus the two interferential fields have important advantages compared with other low-frequency currents, the indications for their therapeutic application coinciding.

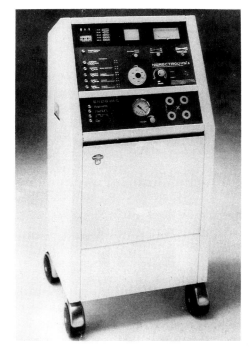

Fig. 1.3 Nemectrodyn-8 interferential therapy unit (FRG).

Modern units (Fig. 1.3)[2] allow for the automatic application of IC of selected frequencies, for example a constant frequency of 100 Hz or the whole range from 0 to 100 Hz at a rhythmical rate, or from 0 to 10 Hz or 90 to 100 Hz. Each of the biologically active frequencies of the current

[1] During the procedure the pointer of the milliampermeter oscillates. This oscillation is typical of the dynamic interferential current.

[2] Dynamic interferential current was produced for the first time with the Nemectrodyn-8 therapy unit.

has its own particularities. Therefore the choice of frequency depends on the aim of treatment. Most units can be connected with a suction unit, which allows the application of interferential current in combination with vacuum massage. The vacuum massage and the interferential current mutually enhance their therapeutic effects. Treatment can be conducted at a constant suction or at 15, 30 or 60 pulses per minute.

BIOLOGICAL ACTION OF INTERFERENTIAL CURRENT

The problem of the effect of different frequencies of IC has not yet been fully elucidated. We will consider those frequencies which are most commonly applied in medical practice and have been studied most thoroughly (experimentally and clinically) by us and by other authors.

Experimental and clinical investigations so far have shown that a *constant frequency of 100 Hz* has a suppressing effect on the sympathetic segment of the autonomic nervous system, as well as an analgesic one. For this reason the frequency is applied when there is severe pain and in conditions accompanied by vasospasm. It is also used as a preliminary treatment in nearly all diseases treatable by interferential therapy.

The effect of a *rhythmical frequency of 90–100 Hz* is similar to that of the constant frequency of 100 Hz, but the rhythm in this case prevents tissue adaptation to the same frequency, i.e. to the same stimulation. That is particularly important because it is a frequent reason for failure of physiotherapy. A *rhythmical frequency of 50–100 Hz* has mainly a sedative and spasmolytic effect.

Frequencies below 50 Hz have a stimulating effect and excite motor nerves, the influence increasing below 25 Hz. A rhythmical frequency of 0–10 Hz or 0–15 Hz is therefore used to obtain movements in articular contractures, e.g. for muscle exercise or to strengthen vascular walls. A rhythmical frequency of 0–10 Hz of suitable dosage results in unsustained muscular contractions, while a rhythmical frequency of 25–50 Hz has a tetanic (Faradic) effect.

What are the advantages of muscular contractions with interferential current? Long-term ad-

ministration of a given drug at the same dosage becomes ineffective. Similarly, when muscle contractions are elicited at a constant frequency, their amplitude decreases and their rheobase increases. Interferential current allows rhythmical change and thus prevents fatigue.[3]

The rhythmical current within the whole frequency range of 0–100 Hz has a predominantly stimulating effect, combined with an analgesic one. This rhythmical frequency often results in active hyperaemia, acceleration of the lymph flow and activation of cell functions, and it enables the restoration of normal tissue reactions, including that of vascular walls. It prompts elimination of toxic metabolic products, dispersion of oedemas, removal of tissue anoxaemia (often inducing pain) and activation of electrolyte metabolism (Ca, K and Na for example).

Some authors have summarised the selective effect of a variety of frequencies in the following way: 'low' frequencies of 0 to 10 to 25 Hz are motor stimulating and cause muscle contractions, and 'high' frequencies of over 50 Hz have a sympatheticolytic effect.

The effect of a rhythmical (i.e. 0–100 Hz) versus a constant frequency of 100 Hz is not strictly differentiated and that of other frequencies is always present. The following effects of interferential current stimulations are accepted:

1. Stimulation of blood circulation through vasodilation leading to improved tissue oxygen supply and rapid elimination of toxic metabolic products.
2. Analgesic effect, considered by the majority of authors to be stronger than that of other electric currents used for therapeutic purposes.
3. Stimulating effect.
4. Selective response of one or other segment of the autonomic nervous system depending on the IC frequency applied; predominance of parasympathetic tone — vagotonic and relaxing action at a frequency of 100 Hz and sympatheticotonic effect at frequencies of 0 to 10/15 Hz.

---

[3] See also the section on histochemical investigations in traumatic neuritis (Ch.2).

5. Favourable effect on trophism by activating tissue functions. Interferential therapy leads to ion shifting, modification of limiting cell potentials, permeability and an electro-osmotic rise.

These manifestations prevail to a greater or lesser degree depending on the type of applied interferential current (constant or rhythmical frequency, type of rhythmical frequency). Thailhades (1959) summarised the effect of IC in this way: sedation of the sympathetic system, excitation of the parasympathetic system and release of acetylcholine in the body.

The first reports on the clinical results of interferential therapy in the treatment of a variety of diseases were made by Burghart (1951, 1952) and Mutschler (1952), and the above-mentioned effects of interferential current have been noted clinically by a number of authors (Ganne, 1976, 1979; de Domenico, 1981, 1982).

Pärtan et al (1953) and Wolff (1956) found that it stimulates acetylcholine production and Hauswirt & Kracmar (1959) proved that interferential current modifies the pH in an alkaline direction. Interferential therapy is assumed to increase the production of other vasoactive substances.

The vasodilating effect was specifically proved by the following:

— measurements of skin temperature (Fiedler, 1960; Nikolova, 1971a)
— oscillometry and oscillography[4] (Kaindl et al, 1953a,b; Nikolova, 1968b,d; 1971a)
— capillaroscopy (Pärtan et al, 1953; Nikolova & Ivanov, 1974)
— rheography (see Glossary) and arteriography (Kaindl, 1953; Thailhades, 1959; Nikolova, 1980)
— measurement of pulse wave rate and the tensogram image using the Syncardon apparatus.[5]

The effect was proved in patients with obliterating endarteritis and bone fractures (Nikolova, 1968b,d; 1979). Improvement in the pulse wave rate and the tensogram image can be accounted for not only by decrease or removal of vascular spasm, but also by augmented collateral circulation. After blockade of the cervico-thoracic ganglion with interferential current a vasodilating effect was also observed in patients with no response to sympathectomy (Burghart, 1952; Nikolova, 1969d,e, 1971a).

Both clinically and experimentally interferential therapy has been found to stimulate regeneration of damaged peripheral nerves and to improve muscle function. For instance Pärtan et al (1953) and Fiedler (1960), having defined the rheobase, accommodation coefficient and intensity-time curves, proved that interferential therapy helps to normalise these indices. They found that the extent of improvement in accommodation depends on the therapeutic field size, and also that improvement in electro-excitability is observed both in the treated and in the unaffected opposite side. This gave them grounds for accepting the presence of a certain remote influence in a neuro-reflex way. Using classical methods of diagnosis (old Faradic, Galvanic test — see Glossary) it was found that in peripheral nerve damage, interferential current at a rhythmical frequency between 0–100 Hz results in improvement of pathological changes in electro-excitability (Nikolova, 1966a, 1971a). The same positive effect was also proved by means of electromyography (Nikolova, 1973b).

Clinical and radiological observations over the period 1963 to 1969 showed that IT stimulates both endosteal and periosteal callus formation (Nikolova, 1969f) and that metal implants are not a contraindication in interferential therapy. This was confirmed experimentally later by Laabs (1982a,b).

Burghart (1952) claims that interferential current possesses certain bactericidal properties similar to those of short wave and ultrasound. He believes that this accounts for its positive effect on purulent processes in the middle ear, for example. The data have not been confirmed by other authors. However, beneficial effect has been observed in traumatic chronic osteomyelitis (Nikolova, 1969e, 1971a).

---

[4] On the basis of 800 oscillographic recordings the vasodilating effect was found to manifest itself not only in the area under treatment, but also in the symmetrical unaffected extremity.
[5] Swiss-made apparatus for syncardial massage (see Glossary)

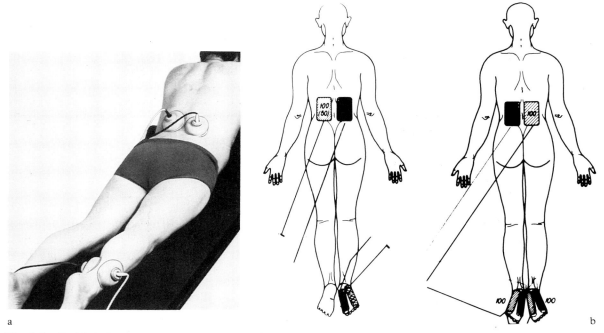

a

b

Fig. 1.4 a. Position of electrodes in sciatica. b. Position of electrodes in simultaneous treatment of the two extremities.

INTERFERENTIAL THERAPY: TECHNIQUE AND METHODS

Interferential current is applied through metal electrodes placed in viscose pads in the following way:

The body part to be treated is encircled by 4-plate electrodes in such a fashion that the two medium-frequency currents cross in it (Fig. 1.4a). The size of the electrodes is selected depending on the affected area — 200, 100, 50 cm^2 or less. If the action is to be enhanced in an area proximal to the back half of the body, electrodes of a smaller size are positioned dorsally, and the larger ones ventrally. If the two lower extremities are subject to simultaneous treatment, 6 electrodes (Fig 1.4b) are applied, using a connecting wire. The distance between the electrodes and the affected area can vary, but the electrodes should never come in contact with each other and should be placed on soft tissue and not on bony areas.

Before each application the skin should be cleansed of contact medium, if ultrasound was applied immediately before. The electrodes should be firmly bound to the skin, but not too tightly as this may disturb blood circulation and interfere with the desirable therapeutic effect.

Several types of special electrodes have been designed so far[6] and are currently in use:

1. Pad electrodes for surface effect: 1 flat pad incorporating 4 round electrodes mounted diagonally is fixed with a band. This type of electrode is appropriate for the treatment of facial nerve palsy and some skin diseases.
2. Pad electrodes T-red (Nemectrodyn terminology) for action in depth: 2 flat pads which must be applied together in such a manner that the area to be treated lies between them. They are used when 4 small plate electrodes cannot be positioned or this is inappropriate, for instance in occipital neuralgia. They are placed transversally when used for treatment of the small joints of the fingers. When placed longitudinally, they can produce a superficial effect, for example in superficial small haematomata.

[6] Nemectrodyn 8 apparatus.

3. Four-field electrodes: 1 flat pad (170×170 mm) incorporating 4 flat electrodes which are placed diagonally. This is convenient for the superficial treatment of larger body areas, for instance the back (Fig. 1.5).
4. Two-field double pad electrodes: 1 pair of flat pads incorporating 2 electrodes each (Fig. 1.6). This is applied only in pairs, for instance when the whole spine is to be treated.
5. Electrodes for the mammary glands: they are ring-like in shape and are aimed at stimulating lactation, as well as strengthening the loosened muscle tissues.
6. Ocular electrodes (Fig. 1.7): they are adapted to act upon the brain.
7. Glove electrodes.
8. Four-point electrodes: for treatment of small areas and for electro-acupuncture with interferential current (Fig. 1.8).

When interferential current and vacuum massage are applied simultaneously, pulsed suction is indicated. Rubber or plastic cups of different sizes are applied, each electrode plate being fixed inside. They are easily fixed to the body and can be adjusted to its shape. It has been found that pulsed suction stimulates circulation and allows better transport of tissue fluids than if interferential current is used in isolation.

The intensity of the current selected in IT depends on the electrode area (objective criterion) and on the individual sensitivity of the patient (subjective criterion). The average dose is within the range of 4 to 50 mA. The patient should experience a sensation of deep, sufficiently strong, but pleasantly vibrating massage at rhythmical frequencies and a pleasant tingling sensation at a constant frequency of 100 Hz. It should be borne in mind that at 'higher frequencies' (constant frequency of 100 Hz and rhythmical frequency of 90–100 Hz) patients can as a rule tolerate a higher intensity of current than at lower frequencies, especially from 0–10 Hz. As soon as the initial dosage is selected, it can be increased only once if the patient's sensation of the current has weakened or disappeared. The patient should actively participate in determining the dosage after he has

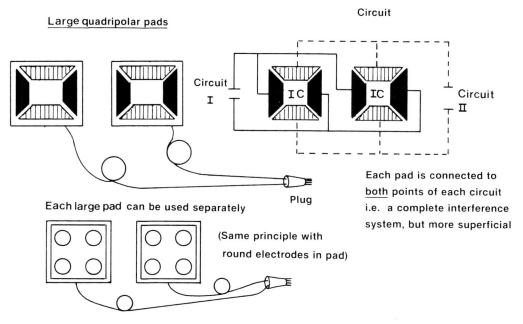

Quadripolar arrangement
4–field electrode

Large quadripolar pads

Circuit

Circuit
I

IC   IC

Circuit
II

Each large pad can be used separately

Plug

(Same principle with round electrodes in pad)

Each pad is connected to both points of each circuit i.e. a complete interference system, but more superficial

Fig. 1.5 4-field electrode — large.

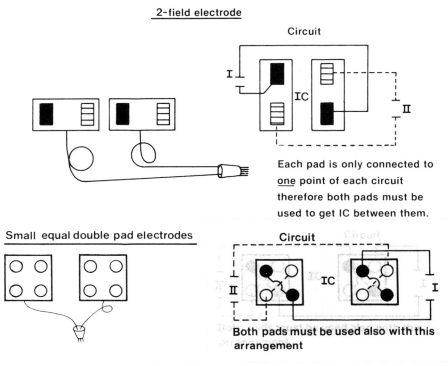

2-field electrode

Circuit

I

IC

II

Each pad is only connected to <u>one</u> point of each circuit therefore both pads must be used to get IC between them.

Small equal double pad electrodes

Circuit

II

IC

I

Both pads must be used also with this arrangement

Fig. 1.6 2 × 2-field electrode.

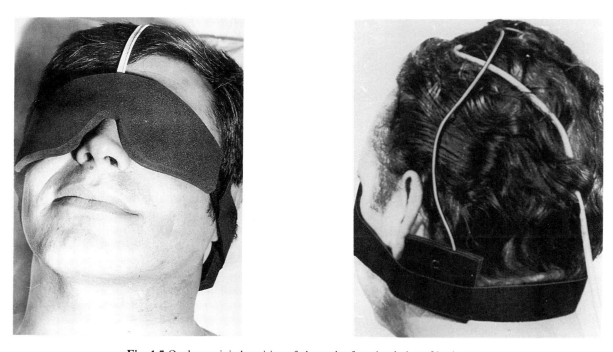

Fig. 1.7 Ocular-occipital position of electrodes for stimulation of brain area.

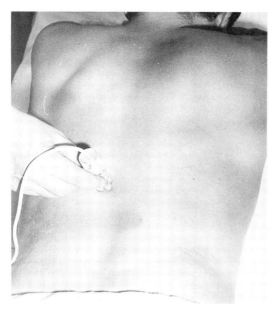 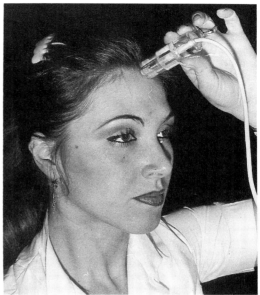

Fig. 1.8 4-point electrode — electro-puncture with interferential current.

been told in advance that the best results are obtained at a dosage which gives a pleasant sensation. The objective criterion should not be disregarded, however, i.e. the possible intensity of the current in mA for a given area of the electrodes. One should also keep in mind the general rule that the more severe the disease the smaller the dosage. And one should not forget that high-intensity current in an acute disease may aggravate the pain. In general, the current should not be increased beyond the patient's subjective tolerance, i.e. the patient should never experience an unpleasant sensation. The dosage, especially in chronic diseases, can be higher, but always tolerable.

Our observations have shown that a patient's sensitivity to interferential current depends on the condition of the nervous system during treatment. The same patient may have a different tolerance depending on his initial physiological condition. For instance, psychoneurotic patients can tolerate a much lower dosage than those with a usual response to the sensation of the current. A basic rule, therefore, is that current intensity should be such as to ensure a pleasant sensation. The effect on patients who are able to tolerate a higher dosage is more favourable and more rapid.

It should be pointed out that during treatment and after a continuous treatment neither irritation nor reddening of the skin is observed because of lack of electrolysis. But when IC is combined with vacuum massage, transitory reddening and slight oedema appear after each treatment in the area under the vacuum electrode similar to that after cupping.

Interferential therapy is given every day or every other day, the treatment duration usually being 10 to 15 minutes, with a maximum of 30 minutes (and in special cases up to 60 or 90 minutes). We recommend a treatment duration of 15 to 25 minutes. Depending on the disease, 2, 10, 15 or 25 treatments will suffice. After 20 to 25 treatments, daily changes in the patient's condition are hardly apparent. Therefore, after the completion of the 20th to the 25th treatment, if recovery does not occur, a weekly break is recommended, and then a second therapeutic course or another type of physiotherapy or drug therapy is commenced. If necessary, drug therapy or another type of physiotherapy can be interrupted also for 10 to 15 days.

During treatment the patient must lie or sit in such a position that his muscles can relax.

As far as the method of treatment is concerned,

depending on the pathological process, the stimulation can be given as follows:

1. Locally (to the affected organs and tissues). This is the most common method used.
2. To Head's zones (see Glossary). This method is aimed at relieving autonomic disturbances such as vascular disorders, dysmenorrhoea or spastic constipation in the thoracic, abdominal and pelvic cavities.
3. To segmental zones. Plate electrodes, or four-field or two-field electrodes, are positioned. The segmental effect can be combined in some diseases with a local approach, the treatments being carried out in sequence the same day or alternating every other day.
4. To the stellate ganglion and the sympathetic chain. This method has been proposed to replace Novocain blocks. A considerable rise of skin temperature from 3 to 5°C as well as a rise in the index amplitude of the oscillographic curve have been established. This rise of index amplitude both in stellate ganglion block and with stimulation methods (Fig. 6.6) was also found by us. The methods mentioned are suitable in treating Buerger's disease or conditions after poliomyelitis.
5. Transcerebrally (i.e. using the method described by Bourguignon) with special ocular electrodes and 2-plate electrodes placed occipitally. Stimulation of the brain can be achieved with fronto-occipital and temporo-occipital positioning of 4 small-plate electrodes. Transcerebral application of interferential current has been found to be harmless and can be used in hypertension and electronarcosis.

ELECTRO-PUNCTURE WITH INTERFERENTIAL CURRENT

This was first introduced in Bulgaria in 1983 for the treatment of some diseases. A 4-point electrode (Nemectrodyn-IV or 8 apparatus) is applied on the relevant acupuncture point at a rhythmical frequency of 0–10 Hz for 3 to 5 minutes at each acupuncture point. Dosage averages between 4–10 mA, depending on the tolerance of the patient who will experience a strong tingling or slight prickling sensation.

Electro-puncture with interferential current ensures a pleasant sensation for the patient and gives good results in treating hypertension in the first and second stage, in cardiac stenosis and in cervical arthrosis. It can, besides, be applied by persons trained in acupuncture point positioning and in the order of application to acupuncture points in different diseases.

COMBINED APPLICATION OF IC WITH OTHER PHYSIOTHERAPEUTIC METHODS

One of the basic principles in modern medicine is combined or multiple treatment, i.e. the application of several therapeutic methods which mutually enhance their effects or complement one another. This principle is also used in physiotherapy with alternating, simultaneous or consecutive application of two or more methods.

As far as interferential therapy and other physiotherapeutic methods are concerned, our experience has shown that the following combinations are appropriate depending on the aim of treatment:

1. Interferential current combined with manual massage (or under-water spurt massage) and remedial exercises.
2. Interferential current combined with syncardial massage (see Glossary) consecutively in one day. This method gives convincing results in treating retarded callus formation and Buerger's disease in the first and second stage.
3. Interferential current combined with vacuum massage gives good results in treating tenosynovitis and osteo-arthritis. On the whole, the two methods can be combined in almost all diseases suitable for interferential therapy.
4. Interferential current combined with ultrasound given consecutively in one day is perfectly suited to osteo-arthritis, periarthritis and Sudeck's atrophy.
5. Interferential current combined with vi-

bration massage (Vibrodyn apparatus). Rapid and lasting hyperaemia is attained, lymphatic circulation is promoted and muscular spasm is eliminated. It is appropriate in osteo-arthritis, shoulder-hand syndrome or discopathies.

INTERFERENTIAL CURRENT FOR INSOMNIA AND ELECTRONARCOSIS

Electrically induced sleep is a method which is free of the negative manifestations of drugs — toxicity, cumulative effect, slow elimination from the body in the case of overdose. Electrically induced sleep with IT is therefore promising, the more so since Kolupaev & Ulyanov (1966) proved that it does not have a negative effect on the patient's physiological condition, and is successfully applied in a number of diseases, for example in hypertension and others.

To induce sleep the ocular electrodes should be placed exactly on the eye-balls, and the occipital ones exactly under the mastoid process (Fig. 1.7). Wet pads are placed on the eyelids and under the ocular electrodes. Müller (1966) recommended the treatment with a fronto-occipital position of electrodes and a current intensity not exceeding 1.5 to 3 mA as being very effective in insomnia, autonomic disturbances, cerebral palsy in children and other conditions.

Electronarcosis, induced by low-frequency pulse currents, even in combination with the routine means of modern analgesia, has certain essential disadvantages, such as sharp fluctuation of haemodynamic indices and unpleasant sensations of pressure and pain under the electrodes. This is the basic reason why one should look not only for the optimal combinations of electronarcosis and drugs, but also to develop new methods of electronarcosis. Sachkov (1966) was the first to propose using IC for electronarcosis. As a main advantage he points to the fact that a current which is less irritating than the one produced in depth passes through the skin underlying the electrodes. An electronarcotic and electrically inducing sleep (EIS) unit with interferential current at a constant frequency of 200 Hz has been developed in the USSR.

Electronarcosis and EIS with interferential current have been studied (and are being studied) clinically and experimentally by a number of authors. The observations of Sachkov & Melnikov (1966) showed that anaesthesia with IC was completely safe in complex and extensive operations, and that it was milder than electronarcosis with pulsed current. Both these and other authors have found minimum side effects with ocular-occipital positioning of the electrodes, and in absence of any appreciable electro-encephalogram changes, as was shown experimentally in animals (monkeys and dogs) and as was observed in humans. Variations in pulse rate and arterial pressure are insignificant and considerably lower than in electronarcosis with an alternating sinusoidal current of low frequency. The actual distribution among the most important brain structures is of greater benefit. Electronarcosis with IC can be successfully combined with drugs and muscle relaxants. For instance IC stimulation was found to be potentiated by barbiturates.

INDICATIONS AND CONTRA-INDICATIONS FOR THE APPLICATION OF IC

Interferential therapy is successfully applied in a number of diseases, and in some of them it is considered to be the method of choice. On the basis of personal experience for more than 20 years we have found that this treatment has proved to be most effective in bone injuries and their complications, in some nervous and occupational diseases and in sterility in women due to unspecific inflammatory diseases of the reproductive organs, in peripheral nerve disease and in peripheral nerve lesions. In the last few years interferential therapy has also found an ever wider application in geriatrics.

It is not to be used in any condition with pyrexia, acute local infections (e.g. carbuncle, lymphangitis), acute and subacute thrombophlebitis, Parkinson's disease, multiple sclerosis and in pregnancy when it involves abdominal and sacral applications, although treatments outside this area are possible and harmless.

PART TWO

Experimental studies

2

Personal experimental studies on interferential current

Many clinical observations are available on the therapeutic effect of interferential current as demonstrated by numerous clinico-physiological tests. However, experimental investigations on the mechanism of action of IC and its advantages compared with other electrotherapeutic methods are scarce. Comparative studies have therefore been carried out by us using an experimental model of some diseases.

COMPARATIVE STUDIES ON THE EFFECT OF IC, MICROWAVES AND ULTRASOUND IN TRAUMATIC LESIONS OF THE PERIPHERAL NERVE IN RATS

Histochemical studies on the influence of IC

There are many reports in the literature on the changes in the activity of acetylcholinesterase (ACh E) at neuromuscular synapses after denervation. Demonstration of changes in ACh E activity is used as a reliable test for the condition of the contact between the innervating nerve and the muscle innervated by it. There are considerably fewer studies on changes in the oxidizing, reducing enzymes and other hydrolases after muscle denervation (Bozhinov et al, 1973). Muscle changes have been well studied on the whole, but there are no data on the histochemical changes in the distal region of the crushed peripheral nerves.

ACh E activity at neuromuscular synapses decreases progressively after interruption and crushing of the innervating nerve, lasting for different periods of time after denervation in the various groups of muscle. It is recognised that changes in ACh E activity set in on the 2nd, 3rd and 14th day after denervation. In reinnervation after trauma of the peripheral nerve, ACh E activity in neuromuscular synapses is most frequently restored by the end of the first month, but considerably longer terms have been reported. When comparing the results of the different studies, it is necessary to take into consideration first of all the kind of trauma, its severity and the position of the lesion, the species of the animal and the type of muscle, the differences and the technical conditions under which the study is carried out, as well as the uneven evolution of the processes of degeneration and regeneration in a given muscle after its denervation.

A characteristic feature associated with muscle denervation is its progressive atrophy. It is well known that a long-term denervation leads to irreversible changes in the denervated muscles, especially in muscle fibres. First a gradual decrease is observed and finally destruction of muscle tissue, which is replaced by collagenous connective tissue and fat deposits. Prevention of these changes, i.e. replacement of muscle fibres with collagenous and adipose tissue, is possible mainly through muscle activity. Many local and general factors have a negative effect on the process of regeneration. Irreversible changes may be provoked by insufficient blood circulation and delayed blood flow to the inactive muscle during denervation (Saitsev, 1976). Immobilisation, extensive dressings and pain are also factors which contribute to muscle atrophy. Therefore, preservation of muscle activity, improved blood circulation and relief of pain in traumatic lesions of the peripheral nerves are important therapeutic tasks. Electrical stimulation with rectangular pulses or exponential current has long been recommended as a method which helps to keep the denervated muscle in good general condition prior to reinnervation, but the problem still remains of how to combine the maximum stimulating effect with a

minimum pain or absence of pain (Gutmann, 1958).

No experimental studies on the effect of IC on processes occurring after muscle denervation are available. It has been established that IC has strong analgesic and vasodilating effects and quickly disperses existing haematomata (Nikolova, 1979). In view of this evidence, we decided to investigate the influence of IC on a crushed peripheral nerve and the muscle innervated by it in relation to their histochemical and metabolic characteristics.

Material and methods

Sixty-three white rats of both sexes were studied. The sciatic nerve in 53 animals was traumatised 2–3 mm distal to its outlet from the pelvis. The remaining 10 animals served as normals. The non-operated limbs of the traumatised animals also served as additional controls.[1] The operated animals were distributed into six groups (see Table 2.1).

Treatment with IC was conducted as follows: two electrodes of an area of 2 cm^2 each were placed paravertebrally in the lumbo-sacral region, and the other two — of an area of 1 cm^2 each — in the distal region of the injured limb. A rhythmical frequency of 0–100 Hz was applied at a dosage of 2–3 mA daily for 10 minutes, for 10 procedures altogether.

The animals were decapitated after slight ether narcosis. A piece of sciatic nerve was taken for investigation below the lesion and the plantar muscle innervated by its nerve. The following histochemical reactions were conducted:

1. Hydrolases — acetylcholinesterase (ACh E), alkaline phosphatase (AP) and acid phosphatase (AcP).
2. Oxidoreductases — succinate tetrazole reductase, lactate tetrazole reductase, malate tetrazole reductase and nicotinamidadenin dinucleotid cytochrome-tetrazole reductase (NAD-H$_2$).

---

[1] The studies were carried out at the Laboratory of Regeneration at the Bulgarian Academy of Sciences (Nikolova & Davidov, 1978, 1979).

Table 2.1 Distribution of animals by groups

Groups of examined animals	Start of the treatment	Number of treatments
Group I	Left to spontaneous regeneration	–
Group II	From the 1st day after the operation	10
Group III	From the 10th day after the operation	10
Group IV	From the 20th day after the operation	10
Group V	From the 20th day after the operation	20
Group VI	From the 1st day after the operation, but treatment of the unaffected symmetrical limb	10

Results and discussion

All investigated enzymes in healthy animals, as well as in the non-operated limbs of the experimental animals, showed equal distribution and equal intensity of reactions. It has been found that in untreated traumatised animals ACh E activity starts to diminish progressively from the 5th to the 6th day to the end of the 3rd week, and by the end of the 1st month signs of restoration of ACh E activity are observed. It becomes normal after the 2nd month, while in animals treated from the 1st day, the neuromuscular synapses show distinctly higher ACh E activity until the 10th day after the trauma (Fig. 2.1). ACh E activity in animals treated from the 10th day after nerve trauma is slightly stronger compared with ACh E activity on the 20th day in the spontaneously regenerating group. No essential changes have been found in treatment begun after the 20th day. No changes in the ACh E activity of the nerve have been established in any of the animal groups.

AP activity in the muscle of animals treated from the 10th day after the operation is strongly positive in a much greater number of vessels than in control animals. For this reason the density of the capillary network of the muscle considerably increases (Fig. 2.1). In animals in which IC is applied from the 10th day after nerve trauma, AP activity manifests itself in more capillaries, which results in a more dense vascular network.

It is generally accepted that, normally, the nerve shows AP activity mainly in the vessels, in Schwann's cells and in some connective tissue cells. Unlike the animals whose nerves are left to regenerate spontaneously, enzymic activity in Schwann's cells appears earlier in the treated animals. Otherwise, this activity is established only by the end of the 4th week.

AcP activity in the muscles does not show any changes both in treated and untreated animals by the end of the 1st week. An exceptional increase in the activity of the connective tissue, macrophagal and glial cells, is observed with the return to normal between the 7th and 10th week in the nerve of untreated animals. The reaction in treated animals has the same character, but is more clearly marked.

The following has been established with respect to studies of the oxidoreductases: by the end of the 1st week a manifest reduction of enzymic activity was observed for all enzymes in the muscle of untreated animals. Striated muscle fibres which are normally clearly visible are not clear now. The appearance returns nearly to normal at the 12th week. No differences could be established in the activity of the oxidoreductases studied in treated animals. On the whole, up to the 10th day oxidoreductase activity is *higher* than in spontaneously recovering animals. With respect to the nerve it was impossible to find essential differences in the activity of reductases as compared with untreated animals.

The results of the present study of traumatised untreated animals show a reduction of metabolic processes in the denervated muscle which first of all refers to the activity of oxidoreductases. After the application of IC, the metabolism of certain components of the injured nerve and of the muscle innervated by it shows a clear-cut tendency to rise. Of basic importance in this respect are the changes taking place in the capillaries of the muscle, which are most probably a manifesta-

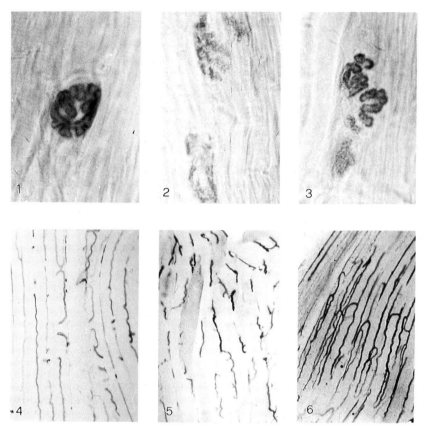

Fig. 2.1 *Pictures 1–3:* Plantaris muscle. Acetylcholinesterase. (Obj.10, Oc.5). 1. Control (normal animal). 2. Ten days after spontaneous regeneration of the nerve — without treatment. 3. Ten days after treatment of the traumatised sciatic nerve with IC. *Pictures 4–6:* Plantaris muscle. Alkaline phosphatase. (Obj.10, Oc.5). 4. Control (normal animal). 5. Three weeks after spontaneous regeneration. 6. Ten days after IT of the traumatised nerve. There is thickening of the positive vascular network.

tion of improved nutrition.[2] This undoubtedly has a positive effect on the trophicity of the denervated muscle. In support of this is the fact that the muscle studied by us microscopically has a bigger volume after IC treatment. Of essential importance is the fact that ACh E activity in treated animals is kept at a higher level. In general, the beginning of reinnervation is marked by the onset of increased enzymic activity, which reaches the norm in treated animals in a comparatively short period of time.

[2] These results correspond to the increased number of the functioning capillaries in the visual field as established by us through capillaroscopy following the application of IC to both healthy subjects and people with various diseases (Nikolova & Ivanov, 1974; Nikolova, 1979).

The process of restoration of the neuromuscular contact is not influenced reflexly after application of IC on the non-injured limb, which shows that the current mainly stimulates tissues with affected metabolism. In confirmation of this is the fact that no changes were found in the activity of hydrolases and oxidoreductases under investigation in the treated intact limb and the controls of healthy animals.

Stimulation of some metabolic activities in the injured nerve and muscle, the first of which is the increased transport through the vascular walls, can probably be accepted as a manifestation of improved conditions for the regenerating process and its earlier eventual completion. The positive results of IT in treating traumatic injuries of the peripheral nerves of various duration have supported this concept (Nikolova 1973b, 1979). It is well known that muscular atrophy often lasts longer after functional recovery (Gutmann, 1958). Interferential therapy is therefore advisable both before and after reinnervation, but undoubtedly preference should be given to its early application, including after operative intervention. The marked analgesic effect of IC is also important as well as its ability to disperse haematomata and prevent the formation of scar tissue.

Histochemical studies on the influence of microwaves in experimental traumatic neuritis in rats

The effect of microwaves was studied in 16 male rats with a body weight of 200–250 g. The animals were distributed into a control group and a group with traumatised right sciatic nerves 2–3 mm below the exit from the pelvis. The group of animals with traumatised nerves was divided into two subgroups: (1) for treatment with microwaves through air (distance 5 cm, power 10 W) and (2) for treatment through a sand pad (power 5 W, i.e. the dosage was decreased by 50%). The radiation in the sciatic nerve area in operated animals started 24 hours following the operation and was applied daily for 10 minutes over a period of 10 days. The same hydrolases and oxidoreductases were investigated as in the group of animals treated with IC.

No noticeable differences were found in the activity of the tissues examined after treatment with microwaves through air and sand. Changes in the control group of animals were absent. This shows that microwaves applied in these doses and with this technique do not exert a manifest influence on the normal physiological and histological characteristics of intact cells, i.e. *on tissues with intact innervation*. Signs of pseudohypertrophy and strongly pronounced fatty dystrophy of the denervated muscle were found macroscopically in injured animals after the application of microwaves. ACh E activity disappeared, a fragmentation of muscular fibres occurred with invasion of round-cell infiltration and connective tissue fibres in the area between the fragments.

The striated character of most muscle fibres disappeared. Infiltration cells showed strongly pronounced AcP activity. Round cells were accumulated in the proximal portion of the muscle where they formed the demarcation line. No AP activity was found in the vessels. The oxidoreductase activity in the injured muscle was completely negative (Fig. 2.2).

These data show that microwaves in the dosage used do not apparently influence the metabolism and the structure of intact tissues. But in denervated tissues they lead to deep and irreversible changes in their metabolism and structure. Therefore microwaves should be applied very carefully or should be avoided in tissues with disturbed innervation.

Histochemical studies on the influence of ultrasound in experimental traumatic neuritis in rats

The experimental studies on the influence of ultrasound (US) on peripheral nerves are not numerous. The histological studies of Speranskij & Svyatenko (1964) have shown that US in small doses applied to injured sciatic nerves stimulates the regenerating process.

No histochemical studies on the effect of US in traumatic injuries of peripheral nerves are available.

We have experimented with 12 male rats with a body weight of 200–250 g with traumatised sciatic nerve. Ultrasound treatment started 24 hours after the operation. Procedures were carried out daily for 10 days. We used pulsed US at a rate of 1:1, a dosage of 0.3–0.5 W/cm^2. The animals were divided into two groups — in 6 of them the procedures were of 5 minutes' duration, and in the other 6 of 10 minutes' duration. We used the labile technique in the direction of the injured sciatic nerve. The same histochemical studies were performed as in the animals treated with IC and microwaves. The intact limbs served as controls, and the results were also compared with a group of animals having been left to regenerate spontaneously.

No differences were found in the enzymic activity of all investigated enzymes in the two groups of animals treated with US, or in the

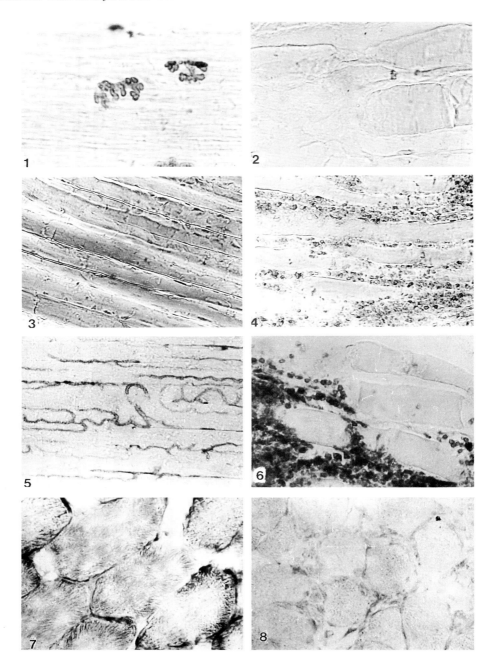

Fig. 2.2 *Pictures 1,3,5,7:* Normally innervated muscle. *Pictures 2,4,6 and 8:* Denervated muscle. 1,2. Acetylcholinesterase. 3,4. Acid phosphatase. 5,6. Alkaline phosphatase. 7,8. NAD-H$_2$.

animals left to regenerate spontaneously without US treatment.

General conclusions

These are as follows:

1. The results of our studies show that denervated muscular tissue possesses various potential reactions in relation to applied physical factors which influence first of all its metabolism. While IC improves the general metabolism of the muscular tissue and greatly prevents its atrophy, microwaves lead to opposite results — e.g. strong decrease in the activity of all investigated enzymes — while US in the dosages used does not lead to visible changes.
2. Interferential current treatment helps to preserve the activity of the denervated muscle until its reinnervation.
3. The data of the present study make us prefer IC treatment in traumatic injuries of peripheral nerves and are in keeping with the electromyography (EMG) studies we have carried out in patients with traumatic injuries of the peripheral nerves (Fig. 2.3).

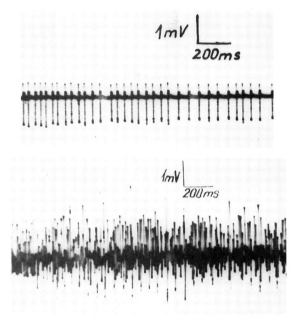

Fig. 2.3 Electromyography (EMG) of extensor digitorum muscle (in lesion of radial n.) a. Before treatment — severe partial denervation — separate action potentials of motor units are registered which at maximal volitional contraction constitute a simple accelerated pathway. (Reduced motor unit activity.) b. After treatment — at maximal volitional contracture a considerably increased number of action potentials of motor units is established composing a rich intermediate model of EMG pathway. (Recovered interference pattern.)

INFLUENCE OF INTERFERENTIAL CURRENT IN EXPERIMENTAL TOXIC HEPATITIS

Research on the effect of IC in experimentally provoked toxic hepatitis has not been carried out. Our experiment aimed at carrying out pathohistological research into liver changes after tetrachlormethane lesion and their response to interferential therapy (Nikolova et al, 1980b).

Material and method

We have experimented with 60 rats of the Wistar species with a body weight of 160 g ($\pm$10 g), distributed into four groups:

— group I (20 animals) with the injection of tetrachlormethane for 10 days, combined with daily IT

— group II (10 animals) with the injection of tetrachlormethane for 10 days without treatment
— group III (20 animals) with tetrachlormethane injection for 20 days and 10 days of IT started from the 10th day
— group IV (10 animals) with tetrachlormethane injection for 20 days without treatment

Tetrachlormethane was injected subcutaneously during the first five days in a dosage of 0.10 ml, and in the next few days in a dosage of 0.05 ml.

Interferential therapy was applied within the liver area on a shaved skin field. The electrodes were placed in such a manner that the two medium-frequency currents crossed in the liver tissues. The electrode area is 3 (3 × 1) cm^2, the intensity of the current is 2–2.5 mA and treatment duration is 10 minutes.

On completion of tetrachlormethane injection and IT the animals were sacrificed and liver fragments were taken for morphological examination. The latter were fixed in 10% neutral formalin included in paraffin and the following histological staining methods were applied:

— With haematoxylin-eosin
— After van Gieson (for collagenous structures)
— After Gordon (for reticular structures)
— After Gomori — PAS — reactions with and without diastase (for glycogen content and PAS-positive substances)
— After Perls (for haemosiderin)

Many mesenchymal and perenchymal alterations were found. More substantial results from the comparative qualitative and quantitative pathohistological studies are given in Table 2.2. Most pronounced from the parenchymal alterations are the fatty degeneration and pigmentation deposits. They are followed by vacuole, balloon and acidophilic degeneration of hepatocytes and

Table 2.2 Comparative pathohistological studies

Pathohistological indices	Groups			
	I treated with IC	II untreated	III treated IC	IV untreated
I. Parenchymal alterations				
Vacuolar degeneration	+ +	+ + +	+	+ +
Balloon degeneration	+ +	+ + +	+	+ +
Nuclear vacuolisation	−	+	+	+ +
Fatty degeneration:				
(a) small droplet degeneration	+ +	+	+	+ +
(b) coarse droplet degeneration	+ +	+ + +	+ +	+ + +
(c) fatty cysts	+ +	+ + +	+ +	+ + +
(d) fatty cysts collapse	−	+	+	+ +
Acidophilic degeneration	+	+ +	−	+
Eosinophil corpuscles	−	+	−	+
Parenchymal micronecroses	+	+ +	+	+ +
More extensive cytolytic (necrotic) changes	−	+	−	+ +
Pigmentary deposits (lipofuscin, bilirubin, haemosiderin)	+ +	+	+ +	+ + +
Initial nodular regeneration	−	−	−	+
Blood congestion	+ + +	+ + +	+ +	+ + +
Haemorrhages and other vascular changes	+	−	+	−
II. Mesenchymal alterations				
Activation of Kupffer's cells	+ + +	+ + +	+	+ +
Parenchymal microgranulomata	+	+ +	+ +	+ + +
Composition of the inflammatory cellular infiltration				
(a) lymphocytes	+	+ +	+	+ +
(b) histocytes	+	+ +	+	+ +
(c) polynuclears	−	−	−	+
(d) eosinophils	−	+	−	+
(e) plasmocytes	−	+	−	+ +
Collagenation of the reticular fibres	−	−	−	+
'Rosette' formation from hepatocytes	−	−	−	+
Reticular network collapse	−	−	−	+
Parenchymal fibrosis	−	−	−	+
Disturbed architectonics (pseudofragments)	−	−	−	+

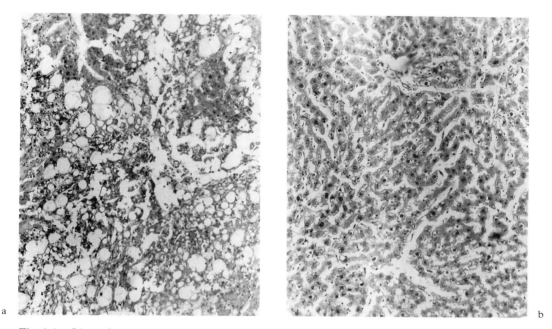

a
b

Fig. 2.4 a. Liver of an animal of group II. Severe dystrophic, necrobiotic and circulatory alterations. Presence of multiple fat cysts tending to collapse. (Stained with haematoxylin-eosin × 100.) b. Liver of an animal of group I. Preserved organ architectonics, enlarged sinusoids. Moderate degenerative changes. (Stained with haematoxylin-eosin × 100.)

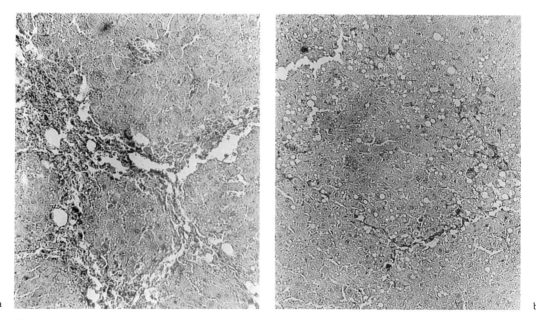

a
b

Fig. 2.5 a. Liver of an animal of group IV. Manifest collagenation of reticular stroma in the place of the collapsed fatty cysts, formation of pseudosegments with initial nodular regeneration. (Stained after van Gieson × 100.) b. Liver of an animal of group III. Preserved reticular stroma, less marked collagenation, moderate coarse droplet fatty dystrophy, restricted in the intermediate areas. (Stained after van Gieson × 100.)

parenchymal micronecroses. With IT (groups I and III) both parenchymal and mesenchymal pathohistological parameters were favourably influenced to a different extent. Most important of those parameters are retention of fatty dystrophy and lack of marked collagenation of the reticular liver stroma (Figs 2.4 and 2.5). These results are in line with our clinical observations on workers with chronic liver intoxication from work with heavy metals (lead and manganese). Clinically, the effect was beneficial. They show that IC helps to improve to a certain degree the functional condition of the liver and to stimulate its detoxic function. The effect of IT in these cases is accounted for by improved metabolism through vasodilation and stimulation of capillary blood circulation.

COMPARATIVE STUDIES ON THE EFFECT OF IC, MAGNETOTHERAPY (LFMF), US AND MICROWAVES IN EXPERIMENTALLY INDUCED D-GALACTOSAMINE HEPATITIS (GH)

The favourable effect of IC established by us in experimentally induced tetrachlomethane hepatitis, encouraged some comparative studies on the impact of IT, magnetotherapy (LFMF), ultrasound and microwaves. As this hepatitis, induced in experimental animals, differs morphologically and biochemically from viral hepatitis and other liver diseases in humans, observations were carried out in D-induced galactosamine hepatitis (GH). The latter was found clinically to resemble liver lesions in humans with acute epidemic hepatitis in its biochemical, morphological and functional features.

Basic objectives of the study were as follows (for further details see Nikolova et al, 1983, 1984b):

1. Reproduction of a model of acute hepatitis in rats to resemble cytomorphologically acute viral hepatitis in humans.
2. Study of some morphological (histological and ultrastructural) liver changes as compared with the serum level of certain lysosome enzymes in the acute and chronic stage and tracing the response of morpho-

logical and biochemical liver lesions to treatment with the above mentioned physical methods.

Experiments were carried out with a total of 100 male white Wistar rats of an initial body weight of 180 g ($\pm$ 10 g) distributed in six basic groups of 15 animals each as follows:

— Control group I — investigated 24 hours following the last injection of D-galactosamine (acute stage)
— Control group II — investigated on the 12th day after the last injection of D-galactosamine (chronic stage)
— Group III — with D-galactosamine-induced hepatitis, investigated after 12 daily procedures with IC
— Groups IV, V and VI — as in group III, but treated with magnetotherapy, US and microwaves respectively; 10 healthy untreated animals used as controls

The liver injury was produced via preliminary threefold (i.e. on three consecutive days) intraperitoneal injection of D-galactosamine (Merck) in a single dose of 400 mg/kg body weight.

Interferential current was applied with the electrodes being located on a shaved skin area so that the crossing of the two medium-frequency currents took place within the liver tissue. The size of the electrodes was 3 cm × 1 cm, the intensity of the current was 2–2.5 mA, administered at a rhythmical frequency of 0–100 Hz for 10 minutes, for a total of 12 treatments.

Magnetotherapy was provided in the following fashion: both inductors were applied on the skin across the liver region in close contact to the skin. Treatment was applied at the rate of 8 mT, at a pulse regime 2:2 daily for 10 minutes, for a total of 12 procedures.

Ultrasound was applied in the liver area on shaved skin using the labile technique at a constant intensity of 0.2–0.3 W/cm² for 6 minutes daily (TUR-US 6 unit, diameter of treatment head 1 cm).

Microwave therapy was given via a portable Radarmed unit (FRG) with a power supply of 25 W; the transducer with a diameter of 3.5 cm was closely fixed to the bare skin of the hepatic area, in a dosage of 2 W; the duration of treatment was 8 minutes for a total of 10 treatments.

After completion of each therapy, the animals were decapitated and liver and blood samples were taken for investigation. The following staining methods were applied for the histological investigation:

— with haematoxylin-eosin after van Gieson along with Holusha's modification
— after Gomori (the PAS-reaction with and without diastase)

— after Gordon and Sweet (impregnation for articular filaments)
— with Sudan-III on cryostatic sections of fixed tissue (for fats)

A Hitashi HS-7S electron microscope was used for the examination. The activity of four serum acid hydrolases was determined as indicative of permeability changes of lysosome membranes in the liver: β-N-acetylglucosaminidase (E.C.3.2.1.30); β-galactosidase (E.C.3.2.1.23); α-mannosidase (E.C.3.2.1.24) and α-glucosidase (E.C.3.2.1.20).

Table 2.3 Comparative pathohistological study

Pathohistological alterations	I Acute stage	II Chronic stage	III IC	IV Magnetic pulse field	V Ultra-sound	VI Micro-waves
I. Parenchymal alterations						
Balloon degeneration	+ +	+	+ −	+ −	+	+
Vacuolar degeneration	+ +	+	+	+	+	+
Nuclear vacuolisation	+ +	+	+	+	+	+ +
Acidophilic degeneration	+ +	+	+ −	+ −	+	+
Eosinophil corpuscles	+ +	+	+ −	−	+	+
Parenchymal micronecroses	+ +	+	+ −	+ −	+	+
Extensive cytolytic changes	+ +	+	−	+ −	+ −	+ −
Fat infiltration						
(a) small droplet	−	+	+	+	+	+
(b) course droplet	−	+ −	−	+ −	−	+ −
Glycogen content and PAS-positive substances	−	+ −	+	+	+	+ −
Pigmentary deposits (lipofuscin, bilirubin, hemosiderin)	+	+	+ −	+ −	+	+
Binuclear hepatocytes and mitoses	+ −	+	+ +	+ +	+ +	+
II. Mesenchymal alterations						
Kupffer's cells activation	+	+ +	+ +	+ +	+ +	+ −
Microgranulomas	+ +	+	+ −	+	+	+
Composition of the inflammatory infiltration						
(a) lymphocytes	+ +	+ +	+ +	+ +	+ +	+ +
(b) histocytes	+	+ +	+ +	+ +	+	+ −
(c) polynuclears	+ +	+	−	+ −	+ −	+
(d) eosinophils	+	+ −	−	+ −	+ −	−
(e) plasmocytes	+ −	+ −	+ −	+ −	+	+ −
Initial reticulum collagenation						
Collapse of the reticulum stroma	+	−	−	−	−	−
Hepatocytes 'rosettes'	−	+	−	−	−	+ −
Parenchymal fibrosis	−	−	−	−	−	−
Biliary ducts proliferation	−	+	−	+ −	−	+ −
III. Circulatory alterations						
Blood congestion	+ +	+ +	+	+	+	+ −
Erythropedesic haemorrhages in portal spaces	+	−	−	−	−	−

Results

A variety of parenchymal and mesenchymal alterations were found in the morphological study of the liver. Some of them were focal, others were diffuse. A large part of the changes have undergone a dynamic evolution and show certain morphologically perceptible differences in the different groups. The latter refer both to the nature and to the severity of the lesion, as well as to the surface of the tissue involved. The results of the comparative qualitative and quantitative pathohistological and electron microscopic study are presented in Tables 2.3 and 2.4.

The most characteristic parenchymal alterations in the acute stage of D-galactosamine hepatitis (GH) are focal micronecroses and balloon and vacuolar degeneration. Other changes affect the components of both the smooth endo-plasmic reticulum (SER) and the rough endoplasmic reticulum (RER). SER is most commonly vacuolised, and RER presents as torn single tubes encircling the mitochondria. Common findings are fatty droplets, some of them containing myelin figures (Fig. 2.6a,b).

In the chronic stage (group II) the most common findings in hepatocytes are late lysosomic forms, cytolysosomes and residual corpuscles grouped round the biliary capillary (Fig. 2.6c). Large lipid drops are typical with occasional myelin figures inside. Mitochondria are more numerous as compared with the acute stage of hepatitis. Some mitochondria are of a linear structure (myelinic degeneration).

After IT (group III) some parenchymal lesions were found histologically to have improved: ballooning or acidophilic degeneration of hepatocytes were observed comparatively less frequently

Table 2.4   Comparative electron microscopic study

Ultrastructural changes	Groups					
	I Acute stage	II Chronic stage	III IC	IV Magnetic pulse field	V Ultra-sound	VI Micro-waves
I. In the hepatocytes						
Amount of glycogen particles	+ −	+	+ +	+	+ +	+
Fatty droplets	+ −	+		+	+ +	+
Nucleus						
(a) pycnosis	+ +	+	+ −	+ −	+	+
(b) irregular contour	+ +	+	−	−	−	+
(c) nucleolar vacuolisation	+	−	−	−	−	+
(d) nuclear phagia	−	+	+ −	+	+	−
Endoplasmatic reticulum						
(a) RER amount	+ −	+	+ +	+ +	+	+
(b) structural RER disorganisation	+ +	+	+ −	+ −	+ −	+
(c) SER amount	+ +	+	+	+	+	+
(d) SER vacuolisation	+ +	+	+ −	+ −	+	+
Mitochondria						
(a) amount	+ −	+	+ +	+	+	+
(b) oedema (swelling, turbidity)	+ +	+	+	+	+	+
(c) myelin degeneration	+	+ −	−	+ −	+ −	+
(d) unusual (queer) forms	+	+ +	−	−	+ −	+ −
Lysosomes — amount of						
(a) primary lysosomes	+ −	+	+ +	+ +	+	+
(b) autophagolysosomes	+ +	+	+	+ −	+	+
(c) cytolysosomes and residual corpuscles	+	+ +	+	+ +	+	+
II. In other liver structures						
Activated endocytic Kupffer's cells	+	+ +	+ +	+ +	+	+ −
Parts of cellular organelles and detritus in Disse space and sinusoid collagenous filaments in Disse space	−	+ +	+	+	−	+ +

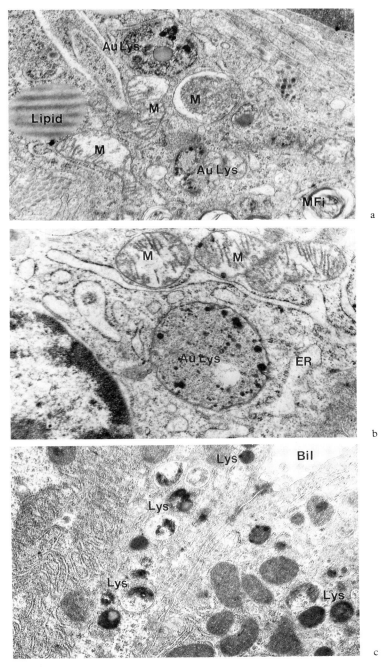

Fig. 2.6 a. Acute stage of galactosamine hepatitis. Oedema and destruction of mitochondria (M), autophagolysosomes (Au Lys), myelin figures (M Fi) and lipid drops (Lipid). (Electron microscopy × 10 125.) b. Acute stage of galactosamine hepatitis. A large phagolysosome (Au Lys), oedematous mitochondria (M), dilation and degranulation of Er. (Electron microscopy × 12 400.) c. Chronic stage of galactosamine hepatitis. A great number of lysosomal forms (Lys) close to the biliary capillary (Bil). (Electron microscopy × 900.)

and the number of parenchymal micronecroses and eosinophil corpuscles decreased. The most salient features of mesenchymal changes are diffuse activation of Kupffer's cells, lack of reticulum collagenation and other architectonic disorders, as well as less evident blood congestion. Most impressive is the increased amount of glycogen rosettes in hepatocytes established by electronic microscopy. A significant part of mitochondria and SER cisternae are normally structured. Typical also is the increased amount of normally structured RER (extensive areas round the nucleus having multiple tubes arranged in parallel) with ribosomes densely attached to them, primary and secondary lysosomal forms and an increased amount of actively phagocytating Kupffer's cells (Fig. 2.7a,b). The amount of collagenous filaments in the spaces of Disse was normal.

The application of magnetotherapy led to the mobilisation of lipids and the activation of Kupffer's cells. Microgranulomas proved larger in size and there was a greater variety of types composing them (macrophages, plasmocytes and polynuclear cells along with lymphocytes and histocytes). Two typical findings were observed using electron microscopy: (1) fatty drops are more common in hepatocytes (Fig. 2.8a); (2)

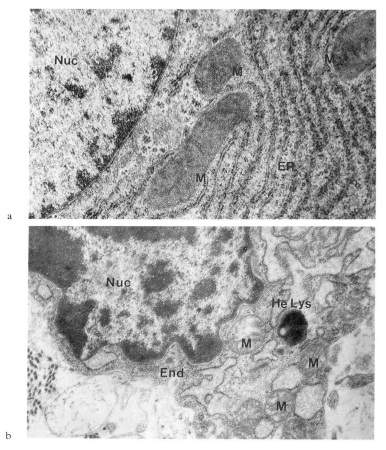

Fig. 2.7 a. Galactosamine hepatitis after IT. Hyperplasia of Er and normally structured mitochondria (M) contiguous to the nucleus (N) of the hepatocyte. (Electron microscopy × 14 000.) b. Galactosamine hepatitis after IT. Activated mesenchymal cell. Spotted chromatin and irregular contours of the nucleus (Nuc), increased number of mitochondria (M), presence of heterophagolysosomes (He Ly) and endocytic invaginations (End). (Electron microscopy × 10 200.)

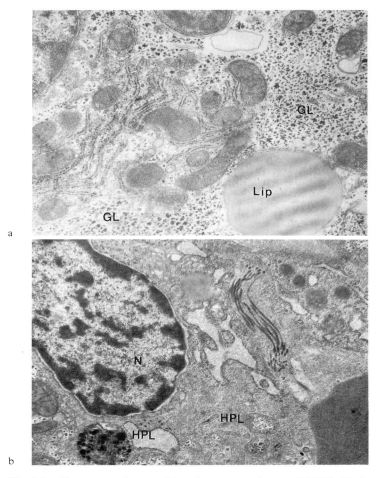

Fig. 2.8 a. Hepatocyte of a rat subjected to magnetotherapy (LFMF). Notice fatty droplets (Lip) filling the cytoplasm. The amount of glycogen (Gl) has increased. (Electron micrograph × 8400.) b. Part of an activated mesenchymal cell in the liver of a rat following procedures with LFMF. A large nucleus (N) with spotted chromatin. Presence of heterophagolysosomes (HPL) localised in the perinuclear area. (Electron micrograph × 7700.)

Kupffer's cells and endothelial cells were more numerous and larger in size than usual; occasionally they were lying freely in the sinusoids, containing multiple heterophagolysosomes (Fig. 2.8b). The latter had absorbed, for example, detrital substances, fatty drops and tubular structures.

Ultrasound therapy does not essentially change the histological appearance of the liver, observed in the acute stage of hepatitis. A higher amount of glycogen particles and fatty drops was found ultrastructurally. Nucleophagia was absent. RER structural disorganisation was less pronounced compared to that observed in untreated animals.

Cytolysosomes and single autophagolysosomes were most frequently encountered, primary lysosome forms and residual corpuscles being comparatively rare. No collagenous filaments were found in the spaces of Disse.

After microwave therapy morphological differences were hardly noticeable compared to the findings in the chronic stage, except for extensive micronecroses, a lower number of activated Kupffer's cells and less marked blood congestion. Using electron microscopy the same changes were encountered as in untreated animals. A considerable number of mitochondria were swollen, the

Table 2.5 Activity of serum lysosomal enzymes (in n kat/l)

Parameters	Untreated controls	Group I after inducing GH without electrotherapeutic course	Group II treated with IC	Group III treated with LFMF (magnetotherapy)
n	6	6	6	6
		β-N-acetylglucosaminidase		
Mean ± SD	764.3 ± 37.2	662.5 ± 91.1	903.0 ± 37.8 p* < 0.05	931.1 ± 33.3 p < 0.02
		α-mannosidase		
Mean ± SD	177.5 ± 7.0	211.2 ± 11.5	248.0 ± 10.4 p < 0.05	174.0 ± 10.8 p < 0.05
		α-glucosidase		
Mean ± SD	152.5 ± 14.4	165.2 ± 11.2	254.9 ± 18.2 p < 0.01	180.3 ± 24.2 p > 0.05

p* – Level of significance in comparison with Group I

amount of lysosomes in the hepatocytes and Kupffer's cells being smaller.

The results of the study of serum lysosome enzymes of animal groups treated with IC and magnetotherapy are shown in Table 2.5.

The analysis of data on serum lysosomal activity and their comparison with the morphological peculiarities of the lysosomal apparatus make it possible to draw some conclusions concerning hepatoprotection achieved by electrotherapeutic methods. Along with the obvious morphological signs of recovery of some subcellular structures and promoted cell regeneration, a well-manifested exocytic lysosomal function is also observed. These are the late lysosomal forms in hepatocytes and the residual corpuscles in close vicinity to biliary capillary (tendency to active excretion of waste products), and in the endocytic Kupffer's cells there are the numerous and variously structured heterophagolysosomes. The results of the comparative pathohistological and ultrastructural observations show that, after IT and magnetotherapy, necrobiotic and degenerative changes in the liver decrease, giving way to regeneration processes. Possibly the most important factor which elucidates the mechanism of hepatoprotection is that regeneration reactions in the liver occur parallel with the increased serum level of lysosomal enzymes and the ultrastructural activation of the lysosomal apparatus. The lysosomal regeneration function is known to manifest itself when cellular defence prompts the removal of a considerable amount of residual products and

biopolymers of no importance. It is in these cases that simultaneous stimulation of energy metabolism and biosynthesis with local enhancement of catabolic reactions are observed. The newly formed primary lysosomal forms, as well as the rapid formation of new auto- and heterophagolysosomes, always result in membrane localisation and an increase of lysosomal enzymic activity in tissues and humoral medium.

The investigations carried out make it possible to grade the effects of the electrotherapeutic methods applied. In this experiment the effect of IT is the most favourable. The hepatoprotective effect here has universal projection on the histological, ultrastructural and biochemical indices under study. The favourable effect of IC is most likely due to improved permeability disturbances and activated functions of some mitochondrial and endoplasmic enzymic systems, with the resulting increase of protein synthesis. Better conditions are thus created for the manifestation of lysosomal detoxication and reconstruction. Metabolism of collagenous proteins and mucopolysaccharides is also likely to improve. Thus the pathological reorganisation of fibrous connective tissue elements in chronic liver injuries is somewhat hampered (Nikolova et al, 1982).

Conclusion

On the basis of research carried out using experimental methods, ultrastructure and cytolytic changes were found rather similar to those observed in acute viral hepatitis in humans. Interferential therapy, magnetotherapy and ultrasound have improved a considerable number of pathohistological and ultrastructural findings to a different extent. Interferential therapy has a beneficial effect mainly on parenchymal degeneration processes such as optimisation of protein synthesis, activation of oxidoreduction processes and retention of reticular collagenation.

Magnetotherapy results mainly in the stimulation of mesenchymal cellular elements which perform endocytic protective functions in the liver. A manifest mobilisation of Kupffer's cells is noted in this group with intensive decomposition and absorption of noxious endogenous products. Compared to IT, magnetotherapy has a less pronounced effect on hepatocytic lesions.

Ultrasound application, compared to IT and magnetotherapy, has a less marked hepatoprotective effect. Microwave therapy in these experimental conditions does not change the findings observed in the chronic stage of galactosamine hepatitis either histologically or ultrastructurally.

The results of comparative studies not only elucidate some aspects of the positive effect of IT and magnetotherapy in liver lesions, but also indicate their advantages. This fact is of great practical importance, giving grounds for the application of IT on patients with infectious or toxic hepatitis, even as early as the acute stage. Magnetotherapy may be accepted to be more suitable mainly in the stage of evolution.

COMPARATIVE STUDIES ON THE EFFECT OF IT AND MAGNETOTHERAPY ON TISSUE REGENERATION

Numerous publications are available on the beneficial effect of IT in delayed wound healing, including wounds due to X-rays and radium rays (Meyer, 1952; Terrier, 1954; Nikolova, 1971a, 1979), but they are based on clinical observations only. No experimental studies are available except for those which show that IT stimulates regeneration processes in lesions of peripheral nerves, established histochemically (Nikolova & Davidov, 1978). Magnetotherapy was also reported to

promote physiological repair. On the other hand, Klouchek-Popova et al (1981) found that some extracts isolated from the blossoms of *Calendula officinalis* promoted restoration of skin and mucous lesions. The addition of the synthetic preparation allantoin was proved to enhance the effect of the above mentioned phytopharmacological substances.

These data prompted us to investigate the evolution of tissue regeneration by smearing the experimental wounds with fractions isolated from *Calendula officinalis* in conjunction with IT or magnetotherapy, using morphological, morphometric and cytomorphological methods.

Observations were carried out on 60 male Wistar white rats (body weight of 200 g $\pm$ 20 g) with surgically induced, standard, circular-elliptical wound defects of the skin of a diameter of about 4 cm on shaved areas of the back under sterile conditions. The rats were divided into six groups of 10 animals each, as follows:

— group I — controls, not treated left to regenerate spontaneously
— group II — experimental controls, treated, with ointment only, containing 5% total alcohol extract from the blossoms of *Calendula officinalis* + 5% isolated flavonoid mixture + 2.5% allantoin
— group III — treated with the above ointment combined with IC
— group IV — treated with the same medicinal ointment in conjunction with magnetotherapy
— group V — experimental controls, treated with placebo ointment (mainly lanolin) combined with IC
— group VI — experimental controls, treated with placebo ointment and magnetotherapy

Interferential therapy was carried out as follows: the electrodes of $1/1 \text{ cm}^2$ were positioned so that the two medium-frequency currents crossed in the wound defect area for 10 minutes, the intensity of the current being 2–2.5 mA and at a rhythmical frequency of 0–100 Hz for a total of 14 treatments. Magnetotherapy was applied transversely through the wound and continuously at 15–20 mT daily for a total of 14 treatments.

The above ointments were smeared daily after measuring the biggest (d_1) and the smallest (d_2) diameters of the circular-elliptic areas. The wound surface (t) was determined using the formula $t = \pi R^2$ at $R = (d_1 + d_2)/4$. Epithelisation in percentage compared to the start of the experiment (0 day) was traced on the 1st, 3rd, 5th, 10th and 14th day respectively, and was calculated using the formula $(t_o - t_n \cdot 100)/t_o$ where t is the wound surface in mm^2 and n is the day of the experiment. The results of the above morphometric studies were processed statistically using Student's t Test and Fisher's Test at $p < 0.02$.

The cytological study was accomplished during the first 2 days, the wound exudate being studied at the 8th, 24th and 48th hour by cell print taken from the bottom of the wound. The cytological preparations were fixed in methyl alcohol and stained after Romanovski-Giemsa with Schiff reagent (for glycogen and mucopolysaccharides) and with acridine orange (for fluorescent microscopy). A biopsy specimen was taken for histological examination on the 10th day. The tissue fragments from the edges and bottom of the wound defect were fixed in 8% neutral formalin, included in paraffin, the staining haematoxylin-eosin methods and methods after van Gieson with Holusha's modification having been applied.

The recovery process traced by morphometric determination of epithelisation rate is presented in Table 2.6.

Within the first 24 hours of the experiment a noticeably stimulated epithalisation was observed under the influence of the above medicinal ointment (groups II, III and IV). After the 3rd day and night during the experiment, the most intensive wound healing was observed in the group which had been treated with the combined action of the phytopharmacological drug and IT (group III). The effect of the simultaneous treatment with ointment and magnetotherapy (group IV) was manifested later. Statistically significant differences compared to the control groups (I and II) were found after the 5th day and night. The application of IT and magnetotherapy with indifferent ointment (groups V and VI) differs substantially from combined action treatment (groups III and IV). On the other hand, after the 5th day and night, the epithelisation percentage in groups III and IV was statistically significantly higher than in spontaneous recovery (group I) and in treatment with phytopharmacological combination only (group II). Interferential therapy proved superior to magnetotherapy, especially when applied between the 3rd and the 10th day.

The results of the microscopic examination have confirmed to a great extent the above morphometric regularities. The cytological study traced the course of the initial inflammatory exudative stage, while biopsy showed the peculiarities in granulation tissue and epithelium regenerate formation. At the very beginning of the experiment certain differences were found in the

Table 2.6 Epithelisation in percentage compared with the start of the experiment (0 day)

$$\frac{t_o - t_n \cdot 100}{t_o}$$

		Stages of observation				
Groups of animals		1st day	3rd day	5th day	10th day	14th day
I	Controls	18.47	30.22	33.30	48.85	79.78
II	With medicinal ointment	32.18	52.98	65.14	78.88	93.22
III	With ointment and IC	39.68	62.26	81.99	89.43	90.04
IV	With ointment and magnetotherapy	36.44	54.37	76.81	85.99	99.11
V	Placebo (lanolin) and IT	18.56	30.03	56.97	75.35	91.12
VI	Placebo and magnetotherapy	18.86	30.13	50.65	73.63	97.45

characteristics of the wound exudate between the groups with combined phytopharmacological and electrotherapeutic responses and the controls. In the former cases the polynuclear cells are more intensively stained by Schiff's reagent, i.e. their PAS-positive content is higher; after 24 hours (unlike the control group) mononuclear blast cells are more common, and after 48 hours a considerable number of differentiated macrophages appear with a cytoplasm rich in different inclusions. In addition, fluorescence tests in these groups show more intensive nuclear (green) fluorescence of lymphoid elements. In the control group, even after 48 hours, neutrophil leucocytes are predominant in the wound exudate, and blast cells and macrophages are less common (Figs 2.9 and 2.10). The biopsy on the 10th day in all controls showed a massive leucocytic necrotic torus on the wound surface with fibrinoid deposits. An epithelial regenerate appeared along the wound defect. The former usually consisted of several lines of prismatic cells without manifest microscopic evidence of differentiation. In the groups with combined phytopharmacological and electrotherapeutic action (and most pronounced in the animals under IT), the leucocytic necrotic torus was thin and in some subjects the wounds were almost exclusively filled with *vascularised* granu-

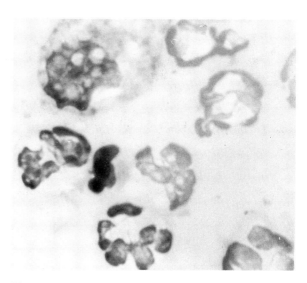

Fig. 2.10 In the group treated with medicinal ointment and IC (group III) differentiated macrophages are often encountered within 48 hours, with cytoplasm rich in endocytic vacuoles. (Romanovski-Giemsa × 1200.)

lation tissue; mature collagenous filaments prevailed; the epithelial regenerate was significantly more developed and consisted of 15 and more lines of cell filaments; the germinal (basal) layer was well shaped and its prismatic cells (often in a state of mitosis) were clearly outlined by the layers lying above, stained in darker colours (Figs 2.11 and 2.12).

Results from complex investigations show that the combined application of IT or magnetotherapy with the medicinal ointment is considerably more effective than when used in isolation. Interferential therapy produces an earlier and more pronounced effect on physiological regeneration and epithelisation compared to magnetotherapy, the action of which is less effective and becomes obvious later in the course of the experiment. The activation of cells with endocytic, clearing functions, as well as the improved microcirculation (Nikolova, 1983, 1984a) are assumed to be of primary importance in these processes.

The problem of how to enhance physiological regeneration is of primary importance. The results of this investigation have shown that the combined application of medicinal ointments with IT or magnetotherapy is to be recommended

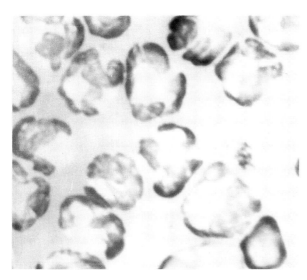

Fig. 2.9 In the control group (group I) neutrophil leucocytes are predominant in the wound exudate within 24 hours. (Romanovski-Giemsa × 1200.)

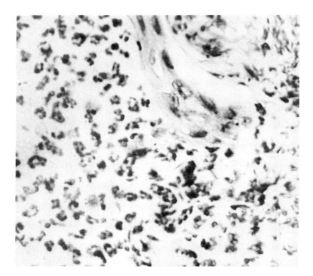

Fig. 2.11 On the 10th day in the control group (group I) the base of the wound was covered with leucocytal-necrotic torus and fibrinoid substances. (Haematoxylin-eosin × 100.)

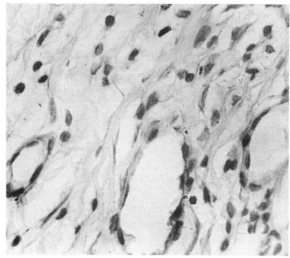

Fig. 2.12 In the group tested with medicinal ointment and IC (group III) the base of the wound was filled with granulation tissue, where fibroblasts and fibrocytes are predominant. (Haematoxylin-eosin × 100.)

in wounds, as it markedly increases wound repair, especially when IT is combined with suitable ointments. Four-plate or two-field electrodes can be applied depending on the wound area and localisation. The former are placed beyond the wound so that the two medium-frequency currents cross in the wound area.

PART THREE

Application of interferential current in clinical medicine

3

Children's diseases

CONGENITAL DYSPLASIAS AND ANOMALIES OF MUSCLES AND TENDONS

Arthrogryposis

This disease is considered to be due to imperfect and incomplete development of the ligamentous, capsular and articular mechanism. The muscles in the area of the affected joints are also very often involved. Typical is the lack of a number of important muscles or whole muscle groups, the remaining muscles being hypoplastic or fibrously degenerated. The spine is spared. The child is able to sit, when he reaches a certain age, but if not subjected to special treatment, he loses his capacity to move (crawling and walking) forever.

The treatment is orthopaedic and physiotherapeutic. Surgical treatment is applied in persisting deformities and contractures.

Rehabilitation must be started quite early. In addition to the daily massage of the affected muscular groups and splinting, beneficial effects have also been attained by IT. It is applied at a rhythmical frequency of 0–100 Hz for 15 to 20 minutes daily, for a total of 20 to 25 treatments. Two to three courses of that kind are conducted yearly, stimulation being given to the affected joints and muscles.

Ehlers-Danlos syndrome

The task of physiotherapy in treating this disease is to strengthen the muscular and periarticular mechanism by suitable remedial exercises, massage and electrotherapy — IC — given at a rhythmical frequency of 0–100 Hz. Treatment is provided daily at a dosage to ensure a pleasant sensation for the child for up to 15 minutes, 15 to 25 treatments in total, 2 to 4 times yearly.

Extension contracture of the quadriceps femoris muscle and congenital dislocation of the patella

These two diseases can actually be considered to be incomplete forms of arthrogryposis or Ehlers-Danlos syndrome.

Contracture of the quadriceps femoris muscle can be complete or incomplete (partial) and is most often unilateral. Adequate rehabilitation measures such as massage, active correction and thermal therapy have to be carried out early and systematically. Interferential therapy at a rhythmical frequency of 0–100 Hz also has a beneficial effect. It is also applied when surgical treatment is required (from the 12th to the 15th day postoperatively) combined with the appropriate kinesitherapy (exercise therapy).

Severe congenital dislocation of the patella is combined with contracture of the quadriceps

femoris muscle. Mild and moderate forms are typical with their special clinical picture (lateral position of the knee cap which in knee joint flexion moves laterally over the outer condyle of the femur). Interferential therapy at a rhythmical frequency of 0–100 Hz is recommended together with other therapeutic methods.

Chondrodystrophia retropatellaris often develops into the so-called recurrent dislocation of the patella. Interferential therapy at a constant frequency of 100 Hz has given very good results in treating this condition (Nikolova, 1971a, 1979). The electrodes are placed so that the two medium-frequency currents cross in the area of the knee joint (Fig. 3.1). Treatment is carried out daily over a period of 15 to 20 minutes for a total of 25 treatments.

CEREBRAL PALSY

Experience with the application of IT in children suffering from cerebral palsy is still insufficient. Only a few authors have reported any positive results, and that mainly in diplegia. Müller (1966) recommended electrical tranquillisation by IC of 1 hour's duration for a total of 10 to 12 treat-

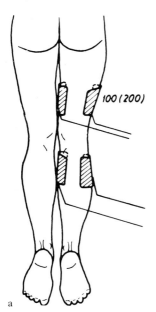

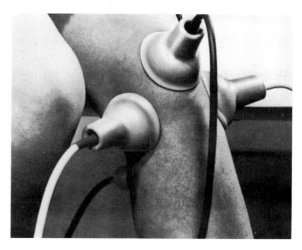

Fig. 3.1 Position of electrodes in treating chondrodystrophy and osteo-arthritis of the knee joint. a. With plate electrodes. b. With vacuum electrodes.

ments. The results are considered to be good. Interferential therapy should be combined with other rehabilitation methods such as kinesitherapy, thermotherapy and hydrotherapy and started as early as possible.

NOCTURNAL ENURESIS

The aetiology and pathogenesis of this condition are not yet fully understood. Two forms are differentiated: functional and organic (for instance lesion of the lower segment of the spinal cord and the nerve roots, anomalies in the development of the spine). Most authors recommend the multiple treatment approach for the functional form by means of drugs, psychotherapy, general strengthening treatment and physio-

therapy (electrophoresis, diadynamic current (see Glossary) and US).

Interferential therapy gives convincing results in treating this condition. It is applied in the following way: two electrodes of an area of 50 cm^2 each are placed in the inguinal folds, and the other two of an area of 100 cm^2 each in the region of the posterior upper third of the two thighs, under the gluteal fold (Fig. 3.2). A rhythmical frequency of 0–10 and 0–100 Hz is applied for 10 minutes daily for a total of 15 to 20 procedures. If necessary, another therapeutic course is conducted after a 15-day break.[1]

Interferential therapy gives positive results in treating the organic form as well, when combined with relevant treatment of the basic disease.

HAEMOPHILIA

Modern substitution therapy in patients suffering from haemophilia has enabled the application of some physical factors such as electrophoresis and microwaves in the treatment of haematomata and haemarthrosis in children suffering from haemophilia.

We have introduced IT, applied at a rhythmical frequency of 0–100 Hz in haemarthrosis patients applied in the same way as in cases of arthrosis of the knee, elbow and other joints. In the case of soft tissue haematomas, the electrodes are arranged so that the interference is localised through the haematoma. Treatments are performed daily for 15 minutes until the haematoma disappears. We have observed that, because of the marked trophic effect of IT, the results obtained from it are better than those from other physiotherapeutic methods.

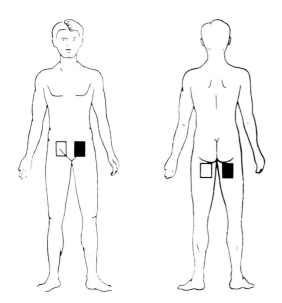

Fig. 3.2 Position of electrodes in treating nocturnal enuresis.

[1] Interferential therapy is also very successful in treating urinary stress incontinence (McQuire, 1975; Nikolova, 1983).

4

Gynaecological diseases

ADNEXITIS

Physiotherapeutic methods play an important role in the treatment of inflammatory diseases of the female reproductive organs. Interferential therapy in treating subacute and chronic adnexitis was proposed by Leeb (1955). He observed positive results even in cases where other physiotherapeutic means proved insufficient, but he did not report data on the effect of IC on patients with primary and secondary sterility.[1]

Sterility

Despite progress in the last few years in treating non-specific pelvic inflammatory disease, the problem of the successful treatment of sterility in women has not yet been solved. The development and introduction of new effective therapeutic methods are tasks of the utmost importance. Having successfully applied IT in adnexitis and parametritis between 1963 and 1965 (Nikolova, 1971a), the author undertook a study on the application of IC in women with adnexal, i.e. tubal sterility. Interferential current was applied either separately, or in combination with microwaves, or alternating with US.

The reasoning behind this approach was that IC, at a constant frequency of 100 Hz and a

[1] de Bisschop (1962) applied IC on experimental animals during pregnancy and did not find any harmful influence on the fetus. However, as was noted earlier, we feel that it is not advisable to apply IC in the abdominal and pelvic regions during pregnancy.

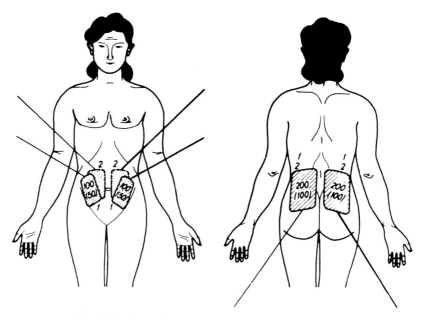

Fig. 4.1 Position of electrodes in treating bilateral adnexitis.

rhythmical frequency of 0–100 Hz, has analgesic and vasodilating effects. It also allows the rapid elimination of toxic metabolic products and ensures better oxygen supply to tissues. In addition it changes the pH to the alkaline side and helps to disperse infiltrations and adhesions. Therefore when combined with US or microwave therapy, IC might be expected to enhance their therapeutic effects.

Interferential therapy was applied with 4-plate electrodes, two of 200 cm^2 and two of 100 cm^2, placed as shown in Figure 4.1. A constant frequency of 100 Hz was used in the first 3 treatments, followed by a rhythmical frequency of 0–100 Hz, the dosage being from 12 to 25 mA depending on the individual tolerance of the patient. The duration of each of the 15 to 20 treatments was 15 to 20 minutes daily or every other day, alternating with microwave therapy.[2]

Microwave therapy through sand was carried out as follows: a round pad with clean, washed sea sand (diameter of the pad 10 to 15 cm, 2 cm thick) was placed first over the left and then the right

ovary and Fallopian tube areas; the round transducer of the apparatus (for example Radarmed) was in tight contact with the sand pad; the dosage was slightly thermal, and lasted for 6 to 12 minutes daily or every other day, alternating with IC, for a total of 15 treatments. Ultrasound therapy was preceded by IT (see above), US being applied at a dosage of 0.2–0.4 W/cm^2 for 5 to 6 minutes first on the left and then the right side, for a total of 10 to 12 treatments. A GDR Sonostat therapy unit was used.

Our systematic observations included a total of 170 women with sterility due to chronic inflammatory changes in the adnexa (Table 4.1) who

Table 4.1 Gynaecological condition causing sterility

Type of sterility	Number of patients
Primary sterility	
with bilateral adnexal changes	79
with unilateral adnexal changes	6
with adnexitis and parametritis	4
Secondary sterility	
with bilateral adnexal changes	61
with unilateral adnexal changes	17
with adnexitis and parametritis	3

---

[2] Treatment can also be carried out with two vacuum electrodes placed ventrally and 2-plate electrodes dorsally.

Table 4.2 Age distribution of patients with sterility

Age (in years)	Number of patients	Conception after treatment
20–25	30	4(13%)
26–30	80	15(19%)
31–35	35	7(20%)
36–41	25	4(16%)

Table 4.3 Duration of sterility

Duration of sterility and previous treatment	Number of patients	Conception after treatment
0–3 years	60	12
3–5 years	44	7
6–10 years	45	7
over 10 years	21	4

had been given out-patient treatment.[3] Before admission the patients had been treated by means of drugs, mud-baths or paraffin applications, KI or $CaCl_2$ electrophoresis, tubs, vaginal irrigations or hydrotubes, but without effect. The age of the patients is given in Table 4.2, the duration of sterility and preliminary treatment in Table 4.3, and the method applied in Table 4.4.

[3] Patients were from the sterility consulting clinic at the Faculty of Medicine and the second City Hospital in Sofia, Clinic of Obstetrics and Gynecology.

The therapeutic effect was assessed on the basis of the following indices: subjective complaints, gynaecological condition, blood picture with differential count, sedimentation rate of the erythrocytes, transaminases SGOT and SGPT, plasma protein and protein fractions, 17-ketosteroids, basal temperature, hysterosalpingography (before and after treatment in 75 patients) and kymographic insufflation (before and after treatment in 65 patients).

All the patients felt that the treatment had a pleasant sensation. Treatment of pain was most favourably influenced with it starting to diminish after the first 5 to 6 treatments. Out of 122 women admitted with pelvic pain and heaviness, the pain completely disappeared in 108 women and diminished in 14 by the end of the treatment.

Other clinical investigations before and after treatment did not show any deviation from the norm with the exception of the erythrocyte sedimentation rate, which was slightly raised in 20 patients before treatment and became normal in all patients after treatment. These data are indicative of a chronic stabilised process on the one hand, and give reason on the other hand to believe that the four methods used do not produce side effects at those given dosages.

The investigation of *basal temperature* before and after treatment with the above four methods

Table 4.4 Response of gynaecological condition to treatment*

Applied therapeutic method	Number of patients	Gynaecological condition		
		Normalised or improved	No change	Conception
Interferential current	82	43(52%)	39(48%)	13(16%)
Interferential current combined with microwaves	53	31(59%)	22(41%)	14(26%)
Microwaves	10	2(20%)	8(80%)	1(10%)
Interferential current alternating with ultrasound	25	24(56%)	11(44%)	2(8%)

* Gynaecological changes on palpation were demonstrated in a number of patients. For instance, in a patient treated with IC a lump as big as a hen's egg completely disappeared, and the erythrocyte sedimentation rate in the same patient improved from 38/50 (after Westergreen) to 6 mm (after Panchenko). In 2 patients treated with IC combined with microwaves, lumps as big as a hen's egg and a medium-sized orange completely disappeared, and the accelerated erythrocyte sedimentation rate in one of them having improved from 25/45 to 3/9 did not show a harmful effect on ovarian function. (This was the first time that the effect of IC on ovarian function was established.) On the contrary, biphasic cycles were observed after treatment (Figs 4.2, 4.3 and 4.4). This is also in complete agreement with the histochemical and electronic microscopic investigations on the influence of microwaves (Nikolova & Ramadanov, 1977; Nikolova & Takeva, 1980).

Gynaecological examination after completion of treatment showed improvement in the gynaecological condition of patients treated with IC, as

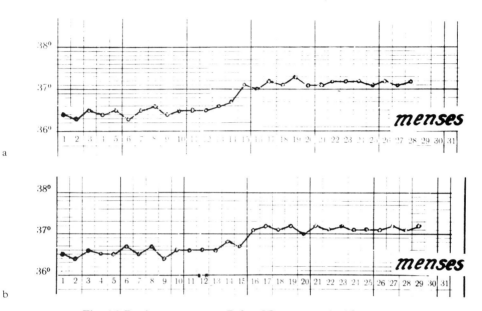

Fig. 4.2 Basal temperature. a. Before IC treatment. b. After treatment.

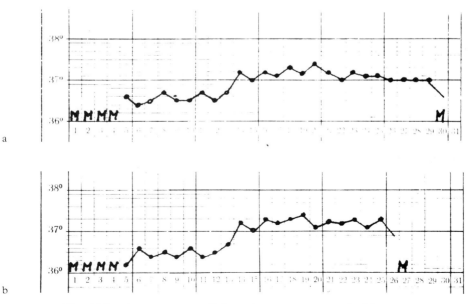

Fig. 4.3 Basal temperature. a. Before microwave treatment. b. After treatment.

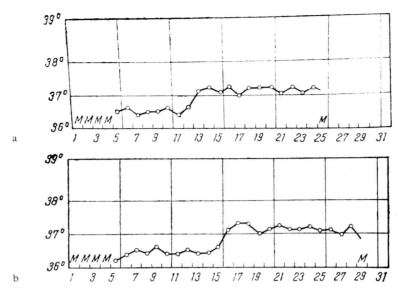

Fig. 4.4 Basal temperature. a. Before treatment with IC and microwaves. b. After treatment.

well as in those who had IC combined with microwaves (Table 4.4).[4] The same applied to the percentage of pregnant women with respect to the total number of women under treatment (Table 4.4). These data show certain advantages of the combined method, which can be accounted for by the mutually enhanced effects of the two factors — analgesia and improved blood circulation and metabolic processes. Bearing in mind that a considerable decrease of blood supply to this area was found by rheography, namely in inflammatory processes in the true pelvis, we consider that the convincing therapeutic effect is primarily due to improved blood circulation and metabolic processes under the influence of interferential and

microwave therapy. The more marked effect of IT compared with that of microwaves (in isolated application) is accounted for by the greatly improved microcirculation and local metabolic processes (Nikolova & Davidov, 1978).

A normalised or improved gynaecological condition was also found by control hysterosalpingography and kymographic insufflations (Figs 4.5, 4.6 and 4.7). For instance, from the group treated with IC in conjunction with microwaves, open tubes as far as the ampulla were found by control hysterosalpingography in a woman with obstructed tubes in the interstitium itself; in two other women with bilateral obstruction, diagnosed by insufflation and hysterosalpingography, the control insufflation showed bilateral patency.

Conception was usually found to occur within the first 3 months, the results being significantly better in secondary sterility (Nikolova & Ramadanov, 1977), as shown in Figure 4.8 and Tables 4.5 and 4.6, but without a statistically significant difference (p > 0.05).

The following examples illustrate the therapeutic effect of the treatment:

[4] Our results were confirmed later by Haag (1979), who recommends that treatment for adnexitis should be carried out with four vacuum suction electrodes at a rhythmical frequency of 0–100 Hz. Treatment in parametropathy is provided with four vacuum suction electrodes at a frequency of 90–100 Hz. He also relates his experience with intrauterine devices (IUDs). In recent years a large number of patients of different ages have been fitted with IUDs. Most patients experienced no discomfort, either at the time of fitting or later. Some patients, however, suffered from acute pain in the whole lower part of the abdomen. These patients were also treated at frequency range III with four suction electrodes. The front pair of electrodes was placed as low as possible in the groin, while the rear pair was positioned in the region of the kidneys.

A 34-year-old patient was admitted with a diagnosis of chronic bilateral adnexitis, secondary sterility. After an induced abortion in the 6th lunar month she had not conceived for six years. Treatment for sterility had been

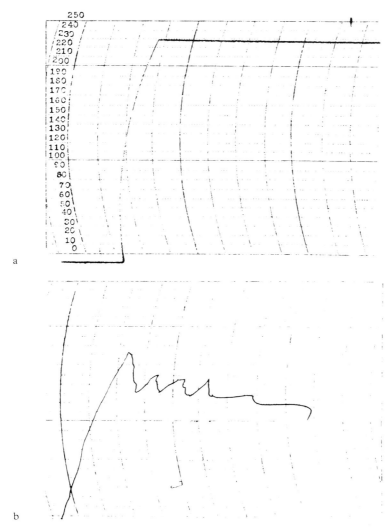

Fig. 4.5 Kymographic insufflation. a. Before IC treatment. b. After treatment.

carried out without effect. Two months after completion of IT she became pregnant, no other treatment being applied during that period.[5]

A 23-year-old patient was admitted with a diagnosis of chronic bilateral adnexitis, primary sterility. For five years she had had primary sterility. Kymographic insufflation showed bilateral obstruction. After completion of IT she immediately became pregnant.

A 29-year-old patient was admitted with a diagnosis of chronic bilateral adnexitis, secondary sterility. For seven

[5] It is necessary to bear in mind that 2–3 therapeutic courses are often required to obtain the desirable effect (i.e. conception and normalisation of the gynaecological condition).

years she had not been able to conceive, in spite of the treatment provided. Kymographic insufflation before treatment showed bilateral obstruction. Interferential therapy led to immediate conception.

A 33-year-old patient was admitted with a diagnosis of chronic bilateral adnexitis, and she had recently been operated on for a retroverted uterus. She had been married for 12 years and had one child who had died. Since 1964 she had been trying to become pregnant, and she had been treated for years for sterility. She conceived immediately after the completion of IT combined with microwave therapy.

The following conclusions can be drawn from the above observations:

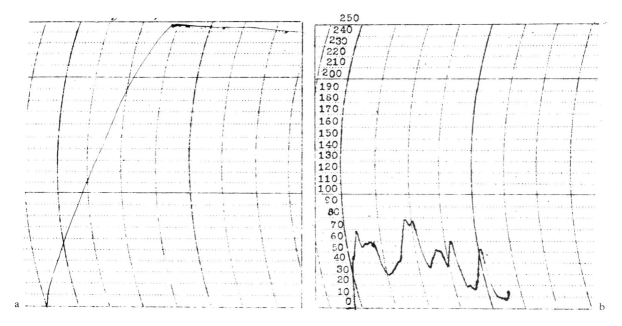

Fig. 4.6 Kymographic insufflation. a. Before treatment, the kymographic insufflation showed bilateral obstruction of the tubes. b. After IT combined with microwaves — normal patency of tubes.

Table 4.5 Conception after completed treatment related to length of time

Conception after completed treatment	Number of pregnant women	Conception percentage depending on time since treatment
Up to 3 months	23	77%
From 3 months to 1 year	6	20%
More than a year	1	3%

Table 4.6 Conception after treatment related to type of sterility

Type of sterility	Number of patients	Conception
Primary sterility	92	12(13%)
Secondary sterility	78	18(23%)

1. Interferential current applied in isolation or in conjunction with microwaves helps both to relieve subjective complaints, such as pain, and to remove or reduce inflammatory adhesions in female reproductive organs. Similar clinical results are also obtained from the application of IC alternat-

ing with ultrasound, but a lower percentage of conceptions is reported.

2. The anatomical and biological results obtained from IT and the application of IC alternating with microwaves should recommend the wide introduction of these two methods in the treatment of primary and secondary sterility due to specific inflammatory conditions of the reproductive organs.

AMENORRHOEA AND DYSMENORRHOEA

According to Leeb (1955) IT gives good results in the treatment of amenorrhoea and dysmenor-

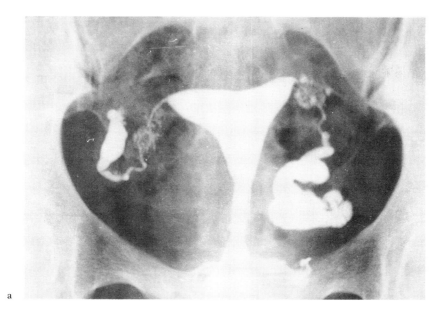

Fig. 4.7 a. The hysterosalpingography before treatment showed bilateral patency of the tubes to the ampullar parts, which are enlarged as in hydrosalpinx. b. After IT combined with microwaves the kymographic insufflation showed opening of the ampullar parts and bilateral permeability.

rhoea, which is also confirmed by the author's personal observations. It is applied in the same manner as for adnexitis at a rhythmical frequency of 90–100 Hz. Some courses in sequence are needed.

PARAMETRITIS

Interferential therapy is applied in chronic parametritis, using the same methods as in adnexitis. It fundamentally improves the gynaecological

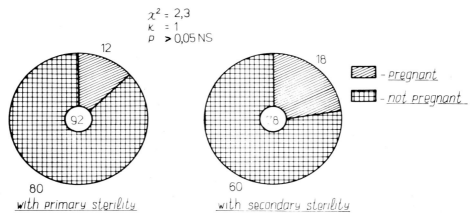

Fig. 4.8 Results of applied therapy using IT in primary and secondary sterility.

condition. The observations of Strougatskij & Kononova (1968) are similar to ours. They observed both relief of pain and essential reduction of adhesions in patients with chronic inflammatory processes in the true pelvis.[6] Further they proved by rheography that IT favourably influences blood flow in the true pelvis, and that this plays a substantial part in the process of healing.

STRESS INCONTINENCE

Interferential therapy for the treatment of stress incontinence in female patients gives good results. It can be applied in the following three ways:

1. Two-plate electrodes, 100 cm^2 in size, are placed paravertebrally low in the lumbar area, and the other two, 50 cm^2 in size, on the inguinal folds. Six to 10 to 15 treatments are applied for 10 minutes daily at a rhythmical frequency of 0–100 Hz and 0–10 Hz.

[6] Burghart reported removal of adhesions by means of IC as early as 1952, and Leeb (1955) noted the favourable effect of interferential therapy in adhesions after hysterectomy, where other methods had failed. It is also confirmed by our observations. The treatment is provided with plate electrodes at rhythmical frequencies of 0–10 and 0–100 Hz, positioned according to the localisation of the adhesions, administered daily for 12 to 15 minutes (with suction electrodes, for 6 to 8 minutes), for a total of 15 treatments. Better results are achieved in combination with appropriate thermotherapy.

2. Treatment is applied as for nocturnal enuresis (Fig. 3.2). Paunova (1972) claims that the patients benefited more from this type of treatment. When urination is disturbed after parturition, treatment is started 2 to 3 weeks later, and in surgical patients, after removal of the Nélaton catheter.

3. Two vacuum suction electrodes are positioned on both sides of the abdomen, and the other two on the upper inner side of the thighs (Fig. 4.9). A rhythmical frequency of 0–100 Hz is applied for 8 to 18 minutes for 10 treatments altogether.

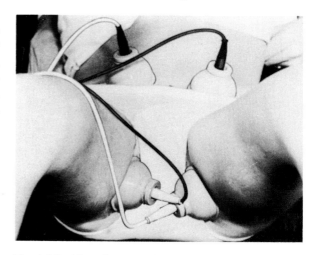

Fig. 4.9 Position of vacuum electrodes in stress incontinence (after McQuire).

The following method has been proposed by McQuire (1975), who has greatly contributed to the use of IT for the treatment of stress incontinence in combination with vacuum massage. He recommends an IC of 25–30 mA (mostly 30 mA), 15 pulses at peak, 0.25 to 0.30 kP per cm^2 (mostly 0.3 kP/cm^2). The duration of the first treatment is 10 minutes; if no unpleasant sensations such as bleeding or backache are experienced, treatment duration can be increased to 15 minutes.

McQuire also combines IT with exercise therapy, stressing that it is necessary to explain its importance to the patient in order to achieve a good therapeutic effect.

It should be noted that IT using the above three methods is not given during menstruation.

Leuthäusel & Rugendorff (1978) applied IT in 43 men with autonomic urogenital complaints but with no clinical symptoms in the urogenital area. They claimed that IT was more suitable than pharmacological treatment. A current of 90–100 Hz frequency was applied in the area of dermatomes T_{10}–L_1. The patients experienced a pleasant sensation with no side effects and the therapy was technically easy to apply. Treatment was given twice a week and the current intensity was selected according to the patient's tolerance.

5

Diseases of internal organs

The application of IC in visceral diseases has not been well studied so far. Experience with diseases of joints, some diseases of the gastrointestinal tract and hypertension is comparatively wider.

THE KIDNEY

Chronic nephritis

Therapy with IC in chronic nephritis aims at improving the blood irrigation of the renal parenchyma. It is applied with 4-plate electrodes of an area of 100 or 200 cm^2, each placed as shown in Figure 5.1. The current applied is of a constant frequency of 100 Hz or a rhythmical frequency of 90–100 Hz. Fifteen to 25 daily treatments are needed for 15 to 20 minutes. Two to three therapeutic courses are recommended yearly. Interferential therapy in chronic nephritis is important only as a component of the whole complex of therapeutic measures.

Nephrolithiasis

Interferential therapy in treating nephrolithiasis has been studied by Egorov & Bogin (1961). It is recommended as an additional method of relieving renal colic (spasmolytic effect) and is applied in the same way as in chronic nephritis.

THE RESPIRATORY SYSTEM

Bronchial asthma

Polster (1965) recommended IT in treating bronchial asthma as an additional method. It is carried out with 4-plate electrodes of an area of 100 cm, or with vacuum electrodes (Fig. 5.2). Two electrodes are placed paravertebrally at the level of the lower cervical vertebrae, and the other

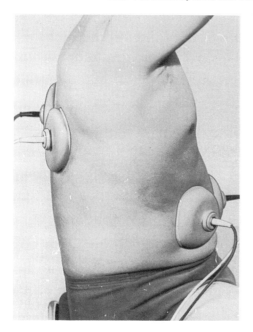

Fig. 5.1 Position of electrodes in treating chronic nephritis.

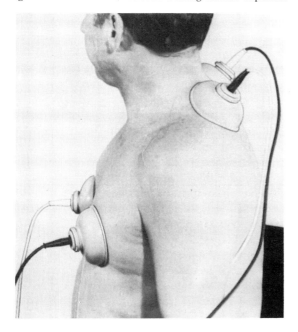

Fig. 5.2 Position of electrodes in treating bronchial asthma and spastic bronchitis.

two parasternally on the chest. A rhythmical frequency of 90–100 Hz or a constant frequency of 100 Hz are applied for their antispasmodic effect. The treatments are carried out daily for 12 to 15 minutes, combined with vacuum massage for 6 to 8 minutes for a total of 15 treatments.

METABOLIC DISEASES

Diabetes mellitus

Interferential therapy in treating diabetes mellitus is carried out in order to improve pancreatic nutrition. A current of a rhythmical frequency of 0–100 Hz is applied for 10 to 15 minutes daily, 15 to 20 treatments constitute a therapeutic course.[1] Interferential therapy is also quite appropriate in treating diabetic polyneuritis and atherosclerotic changes of blood vessels (see p.78 and Fig. 1.4).

Obesity

Interferential therapy is given as an additional approach in exogenous alimentary obesity. A rhythmical frequency of 0–100 Hz is utilised, combined with vacuum massage (the so-called vacokinesia).

THE GASTROINTESTINAL TRACT

Stomach atonia and chronic gastritis

The purpose of IT in treating stomach atonia is to regulate the motor and secretory function of the stomach. It is carried out with 4-point electrodes-T-red-cables (of the German apparatus) which are placed dorso-ventrally so that the spinal electrode is in the T_5–T_6 area and the other is opposite to it. A current of a rhythmical frequency of 0–100 Hz is used for 10 to 15 minutes daily for a total of 15 to 20 or more treatments.

Interferential therapy in the treatment of hypo-acidic and hyper-acidic chronic gastritis is applied in combination with adequate drug and dietetic treatment. It helps to relieve pain and dyspeptic phenomena and to improve the nutri-

[1] Interferential therapy is similarly applied in the treatment of pancreatitis (Fig. 5.3).

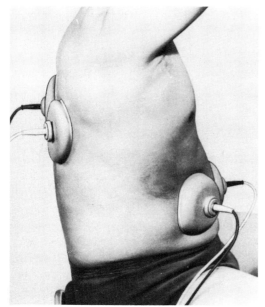

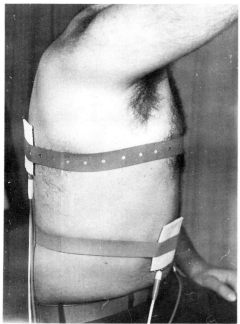

a

b

Fig. 5.3 Position of electrodes in treating pancreatitis.
a. With vacuum electrodes. b. With plate electrodes.

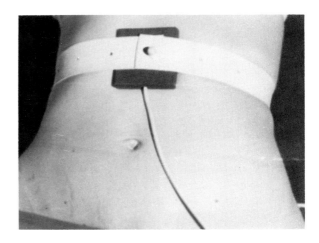

Fig. 5.4 Position of 2 × 2-field electrodes in treating stomach atonia and chronic gastritis.

rhythmical frequency of 0–100 Hz. A total of 15 to 20 treatments are applied daily for 10 to 15 minutes.

Peptic ulcer

Interferential therapy has been used successfully for the treatment of peptic ulcer, provided there is no haemorrhage. It helps not only to relieve or reduce pain and other symptoms of the disease, but also to improve tissue trophicity. Treatment is carried out with 4-plate electrodes of an area of 50 cm² or vacuum electrodes. When plate electrodes are applied, the treatment duration is 10 to 15 minutes; with vacuum electrodes, i.e. in combination with vacuum massage, it is 6 to 8 minutes. The current is of a rhythmical frequency of 90–100 Hz and 0–100 Hz. The therapeutic course requires a total of 15 to 20 treatments.

Constipation

Fiedler (1960), de Bisschop (1962) and others report positive results when IT is used in treating atonic and spastic constipation.

Treatment of spastic constipation is carried out in the following way: 2-plate electrodes of an area of 100 or 200 cm² are positioned paravertebrally from T_5 downwards, and two others of the same size are positioned anteriorly low on the abdomen (Fig. 5.5). A current of a constant frequency of

tion of the mucous membrane of the stomach. It is carried out in the same way as for stomach atonia (Fig. 5.4), but during the first 3 to 5 treatments a current of a rhythmical frequency of 90–100 Hz is applied, followed by a current of a

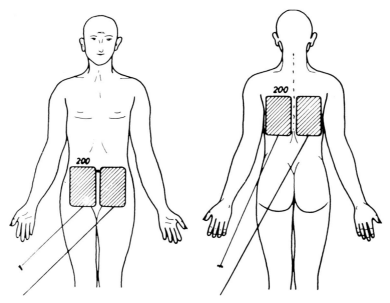

Fig. 5.5 Position of electrodes in treating spastic constipation.

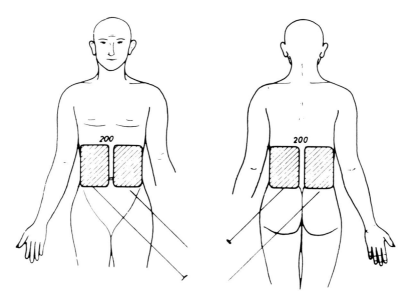

Fig. 5.6 Position of electrodes in treating atonic constipation.

100 Hz or a rhythmical frequency of 90–100 Hz is applied. The treatments are conducted daily for 15 to 20 minutes for a total of 6 to 10 treatments. Some authors report clinical and radiographic improvement in more than half the patients who were suffering from spastic colitis.

Treatment of atonic constipation is carried out with the electrodes positioned as shown in Figure 5.6. A current of a rhythmical frequency of 0–100 Hz is applied for 15 to 20 minutes for the required 10 to 12 treatments. IT using the dynamic field is preferable. The combination of IT with vacuum massage gives very good results. Treatment duration in this case is short — 6 to 8 minutes only.

THE CARDIOVASCULAR SYSTEM

Hypertension

It is well known that a number of physical factors (e.g. electrophoresis, diadynamic current, microwaves, magnetotherapy, different mineral baths, etc.) and electrically induced sleep give good results in treating hypertension in the first and second stage. Electrically induced sleep with pulsed currents was found to have a favourable influence in the earlier stage of the disease.

Electrically induced sleep with IC for the treatment of hypertension was first applied by Putan (1966). He gave preference to IT because of a number of advantages, such as smoother haemodynamics and lack of discomfort under the electrodes. The treatment is applied with the ocular-occipital positioning of the electrodes, at a current intensity of 2–6 mA. A current of a constant frequency of 200 Hz is supplied by a unit designed for this purpose in the USSR. Patients report that electrically induced sleep by interferential current does not produce pain and is accompanied sometimes by a pleasant sensation of being rocked. Improvement was found in all patients, manifesting itself in reduction of subjective complaints, improved sleep and fall of arterial pressure. Muller (1966) recommended that this technique using IC should be applied with a fronto-occipital positioning of the electrodes.

Egorov & Bogin (1961) applied IT in the area of the sympathetic trunk to reduce peripheral autonomic tone and to improve blood circulation. They claim that patients in the first and second stage of hypertension, for whom drug therapy had proved inefficient, benefited from IT.

Electro-acupuncture with IC in treating patients with hypertension was introduced by us in Bulgaria in 1983. The following acupuncture points were acted upon: GV 24, GV 22, GV 20, GV 19 and GV 18. A total of 10 treatments were used with a 4-point electrode at a rhythmical frequency of 0–10 Hz for 3 minutes for each acupuncture point. As a result of the treatment, subjective complaints disappeared or were reduced and the arterial blood pressure returned to normal. This enabled us to stop (for some time) or reduce the dosage of hypotensive drugs which had been prescribed to keep up the favourable

effect. Treatment was repeated after a break of 7 to 10 days.

Hemiplegia

Physiotherapeutic methods which favourably influence contractures of central origin are not numerous. Interferential therapy in treating post-hemiplegic contractures was introduced by Bernard et al in 1955 on the following grounds:

— The ability of IC to produce stimuli localised in depth and to reduce exteroreceptive irritation to a minimum.
— The proven relaxing properties of IC in joint rigidity of traumatic origin using intensities below the muscle contraction threshold.

The authors have treated the upper limb in two ways:

1. 4-plate electrodes positioned in such a manner that they encircle the whole upper limb
2. By blocking the stellate ganglion (see p.98, Raynaud's disease)

As they observed only a slight effect on the contractures using the first method, they later started applying only the second method, which was also recommended by other authors (e.g. Joutard, 1959). They stress that the patient experiences warming of the face and of the other upper extremity during the treatments. Objectively, a slight miosis was observed during the block with a rise in skin temperature of 1–2°C and a slight fall of the rheobase.

They noted that, firstly, reduction of the spastic position of the elbow joint takes place, then, secondly, the wrist and finally the shoulder joint. Sometimes the treatment of the upper extremity favourably influences the lower extremity as well. The authors recommend that the treatment should be continued until the spasticity almost completely disappears. A second stage of the treatment involves local stimulation of the extremities but with 2-field electrodes positioned in such a manner that the effect of the current is concentrated on the extensors.

Gallin (1959), on the basis of observations of

200 patients with hemiplegia, also reported beneficial results from IT. Thailhades (1959) observed 60 patients over a period of six years and found more or less reduced spastic contractures, removal of aphasia and improvement in gait in all patients.

Interferential therapy to block the stellate ganglion was applied by us in 10 patients with hemiparesis after haemorrhagic insult with the same results as described by the above-mentioned authors. This treatment is therefore considered by us to have good prospects and should be provided to patients suffering from hemiparesis and hemiplegia who require rehabilitation.

THE LIVER AND BILE DUCTS

Chronic hepatitis

Interferential therapy in treating liver and biliary diseases (chronic hepatitis, cholecystitis, pericholecystitis) was first applied by Burghart (1952). No reports are available on the effect of IC in chronic toxic hepatitis of exogenous nature. It is well known that the problem of the treatment of the disease is still unsolved in spite of the dietary cures and the variety of drugs and physiotherapeutic methods applied and proposed.

Hepatotoxic substances are considered to disturb the normal metabolic chains in fat, protein and carbohydrate metabolism. Interferential current has been shown to have both analgesic and vasodilating effects, to improve metabolism and to help tissue trophicity return to normal. The basic purpose of each type of treatment in exogenous toxic hepatitis is to enhance the detoxicating function of the liver and to activate the repair processes in order to prevent chronic hepatitis developing into cirrhosis. By the mechanism of its action IT meets these requirements. It was introduced by us as a therapeutic method for the treatment of the disease in 1976–1977.

Observations were made on 33 patients with chronic intoxication and lesion of the liver who had been working with heavy metals (lead, manganese). They were aged between 20 and 57 years and included 32 men and 1 woman. Thirty had chronic persisting hepatitis and 3 patients had compensated liver cirrhosis. The patients' symptoms are given in Table 5.1.

Interferential therapy was applied with 4-plate electrodes of an area of 150 cm^2 placed so as to enable the liver to be in the interference area of the two medium-frequency currents (Fig. 5.7). A current of a constant frequency of 100 Hz was applied in the first 3 treatments, and a rhythmical frequency of 0–100 Hz in the others, daily for 15 to 20 minutes, for a total of 15 to 25 treatments.

The subjective complaints of the patients were favourably influenced by the therapy and the hepatomegaly diminished by 1–2 cm. The urine analysis (albumin, bilirubin, urobilinogen) before and after treatment did not show any deviations from the norm. The leukocyte count, blood sugar and sedimentation test before and after treatment were also within normal limits (the sedimentation rate was slightly accelerated in only 2 patients, returning to normal after the treatment). The haemoglobin proved to be slightly decreased in 8 patients, but a statistically significant ($p < 0.05$) tendency to rise was noted (before treatment Hb = 13.55 + 1.630, after treatment Hb = 14.544 + 1.558). Increased serum bilirubin was found in 2 patients with persisting hepatitis (1.06 and 1.35 mg%) with its normalisation after the treatment. The plasma protein level in 5 patients was slightly

Table 5.1 Symptoms of patients with chronic hepatitis

Symptoms	Number of patients		
	Symptoms before treatment	Disappeared or diminished symptoms	Unchanged symptoms
Pain in the right hypochondrium	33	30(90%)	3
Dyspeptic complaints	33	28(85%)	5
Hepatomegaly	27	19(70%)	8
Hepatosplenomegaly	3	1(33%)	2

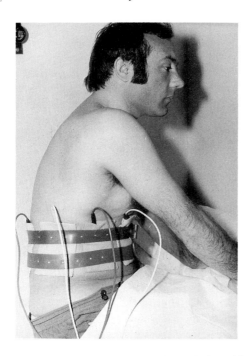

Fig. 5.7 Position of electrodes in treating toxic hepatitis.

increased before the treatment. The same applied to the total cholesterol. There were 6 patients with deviation in the thymol turbidity test, the test becoming normal in 5 of them after treatment. The changes in all these indices are statistically insignificant ($p > 0.05$). The same applies to Weltmann's flocculation reaction. Blood histamine levels were examined in 24 patients after Rosenthal-Tabor's method. At an adopted norm of 7–9 mg%, before treatment it proved to be decreased in 10 patients ($H\bar{x} = 5.04$ + 0.83) becoming normal after treatment ($H\bar{x} = 7.45 + 2.07$), the difference being statistically significant ($p < 0.05$). Increased histamine level was found in 6 patients ($H\bar{x} = 11.91 + 1.47$) with a tendency to normalisation after the treatment ($H\bar{x} = 9.25 + 1.67$).

The changes in the indices examined show that IT helps not only to relieve or to diminish pain and dyspeptic complaints, but also to obtain some improvement in liver function and stimulate its detoxicating function. These findings are in agreement with our studies on experimental toxic hepatitis in which the hepatoprotective effect of interferential current was also proved by means of electronic-microscopic investigations (Nikolova et al, 1982). The beneficial effect of IT may be explained through the improved metabolism of liver tissue by means of vasodilation and stimulation of capillary blood circulation.

Biliary dyskinesia

Interferential therapy finds application in the spastic form of dyskinesia to control the spasm of the gall-bladder and sphincter. IT is carried out as in chronic hepatitis with the application of a constant frequency of 100 Hz (antispasmodic and pain-sedating effect) as an aid to drug therapy.

Chronic cholecystitis is also favourably influenced by IT, carried out according to the method described on page 57 or by acting on the corresponding Head's zones (see Glossary) with 4- or 2-field electrodes, or plate electrodes in the region of T_8–T_{10}. The aim is to relieve spasm and pain.

6
Diseases of joints

INFLAMMATORY DISEASES

Rheumatoid arthritis

Burghart (1952) and Mutschler (1952) first applied IT in treating chronic inflammatory diseases of the joints. Later Thailhades (1959) applied this method in treating chronic rheumatoid arthritis and achieved favourable results in 40% of the patients. Pärtan et al (1953) applied IT in 200 patients suffering from rheumatoid arthritis, using the current alone or in combination with drugs and other types of physiotherapy. Active and passive movements of the affected joints were found to improve, reflex muscular spasm disappeared and pains were relieved.

We have applied IT in the treatment of patients with subacute and chronic rheumatoid arthritis and osteo-arthritis. Pain was relieved and movements in the affected joints improved. Improvement in blood circulation confirmed by rheography and oscillography before and after treatment (Figs 6.6 and 6.7), is considered to be one of the factors favourably influencing the pathological process.

Ankylosing spondylitis (Bechterew's disease)

This disease was described by Bechterew in 1892, but its aetiology has not yet been completely elucidated. Most authors agree that it is an infectious-allergic, chronic inflammatory process. The main purpose of physiotherapy is to suppress the inflammatory process (in combination with drug therapy), to stop the evolution of the disease and to treat deformities of the spine. Ultrasound and systematic remedial exercises are considered to be most useful in this respect.

Interferential therapy is recommended by Polster (1965) as having a beneficial effect mainly as an analgesic. It is given in the same manner as in spondylitic arthritis (Figs 6.9 and 6.10) and arthritis and it should always be combined with remedial exercises. The alternating application of IC and ultrasound gives better results.

Rheumatic fever

Interferential current is used in the treatment of rheumatic fever in combination with other therapeutic measures. It can be applied only as the rheumatic attack subsides to improve tissue trophicity and muscle function (treatment of disuse atrophy). When it is aimed at acting on joints, IT is given in the same manner as in deforming arthritis. First, it is necessary to relieve pain and to improve the blood circulation. A total of 15 to 25 daily treatments are needed for 15 to 20 minutes, the constant frequency of the current being 100 Hz. Treatment in the relevant segmental area is also recommended.

A current of a rhythmical frequency of 0–10 Hz is used for muscular exercise.

DEGENERATIVE-DYSTROPHIC DISEASES

Osteo-arthritis

Osteo-arthritis is one of the most complex and still not completely understood problems of arthrology. The pathological and anatomical changes affect all tissues including cartilage, bone and soft tissues. First, the joint cartilage is damaged, being particularly susceptible because it lacks its own blood supply. Its regenerative capacity is insignificant, and some authors are of the opinion that it does not exist at all. The changes are considered to be due to a disturbed cartilaginous metabolism, especially that of the mucopolysaccharides (Balaba et al, 1974). For that reason intra-articular introduction of drugs containing mucopolysaccharides is recommended.

Osteo-arthritis (especially at the knee and hip joints) is one of the most common causes of joint function disorder. Some authors claim that 90% of individuals over 40 years of age are affected by it, and others (Emminger, 1964; Nikolova, 1971a) that a degenerative process can also be observed in young people, for example ballet dancers.

Two basic forms are distinguished: primary and secondary arthritis. The main aetiologic features in primary arthritis are: (a) disturbance of the local blood circulation — vascular spasm due to various causes; (b) endocrine or metabolic disorders; (c) repeated injuries — not major, but beyond the bounds of physiological compensation; (d) outside factors such as working under conditions of high humidity, sudden and sharp changes in temperature and barometric pressure or a long-standing, strained body or joint posture.

Secondary arthritis is the final structural result of different acute and chronic processes in the joints, such as congenital anomalies, intra- and periarticular fractures, aseptic necrosis, osteochondropathy and infectious processes.

The high incidence of osteo-arthritis in all countries of the world makes it of great socioeconomic importance, and the problem of its treatment is therefore of major concern.

Pain and disturbed movements of the joints prevail upon the patient to see the doctor. Nowadays it is not a diagnostic but a therapeutic problem. The clinical signs, especially the pain, can be alleviated, but the anatomical lesions continue to progress. Herein lies the problem which is still unsolved, i.e. to find out a reliable way to stop this process.

The main therapeutic task related to the pathogenesis of the disease is to relieve or reduce the pain, to improve the blood supply in the area of the damaged joint and to control the progressing restriction of movements and the concomitant muscle atrophy. The numerous therapeutic approaches are divided into three basic groups: medication, physiotherapy and surgical treatment. Conservative methods are aimed at relieving pain and improving or restoring the function of the joints. The prescribed and recommended drugs are so numerous that it is impossible to enumerate or assess them. Most of the drugs have a symptomatic and time-restricted effect.

Various methods of physiotherapy have found recognition in the treatment of osteo-arthritis not only because of their beneficial effect, but also because of the absence of the side effects which are produced by some drugs. However, there is still no agreement concerning the extent of the therapeutic effectiveness of these methods.

Interferential therapy in treating osteo-arthritis was applied for the first time by Burghart (1951), and later on by a number of workers. Burghart observed relief of pain after 2 to 14 treatments in 34 patients with typical osteo-arthritis without accelerated sedimentation rate who had not benefited from any other therapy. Pärtan et al (1953), on the basis of their observations of 200 patients, reported great improvement in 49%, definite improvement in 28.5%, slight improvement in 19% and no improvement in only 3.5%.

We have applied IT in osteo-arthritis since 1963, and up to now more than 500 patients have been observed[1] between the ages of 25 and 77. The clinical diagnosis was also confirmed by X-ray examination. There were 140 patients with 1st stage arthritis, 205 with 2nd stage arthritis and 155 with 3rd stage arthritis.[2] Interferential therapy was given in the following manner: 4-plate electrodes of an area of 50 cm^2, 100 cm^2 or 200 cm^2 (depending on the extent of the affected joint) are placed in such a manner that the two currents cross in the area of the joint to be treated (Figs 3.1, 6.1 and 6.2). A current of a constant frequency of 100 Hz is used in the first 3

treatments, and of a rhythmical frequency of 0–100 Hz in the others. The 20 treatments required are given daily for 15 to 20 minutes.

On the basis of comparative studies in 1300 patients with arthritis of the knee, ankle and shoulder joints treated with IC only or with IC combined with vacuum massage,[3] microwaves, US or diadynamic current (Nikolova, 1965, 1969, 1971a), the following facts of practical importance were found:

— IT influences the lesions more markedly compared to other routine methods
— the percentage of relapses from 6 months to 1 year is lower with IT
— the results from the combined application of IT and vacuum massage are better
— IT is ineffective only in arthritis with concomitant disease requiring surgical treatment (e.g. loose body meniscus lesion)
— in the knee and hip joint arthritis (initial stage, without dysplasia) IT has a more pronounced effect if the local treatment is combined with a paravertebral action in the lumbosacral area using current of a constant frequency of 100 Hz (see spondylitic arthritis) for a total of 15 procedures administered daily for 15 minutes.[4,5]

A basic principle in modern medicine is multiple or complex treatment, i.e. the simultaneous use of a variety of therapeutic measures which mutually enhance their effect or complement one another. This principle is applied in physiother-

---

[1] Interferential therapy was combined with remedial exercises in 100 patients because it helps to improve blood supply and maintain tissue elasticity although these exercises are contra-indicated in marked local inflammatory phenomena. In principle, general strengthening exercises are applied as well as special ones for the damaged joint. They are planned individually according to the age, training and general condition of the patient, and the condition of the affected joints. The exercises are carried out without physical effort, so as not to traumatise the affected tissues.

[2] *1st stage arthritis* Clinical data (symptoms) are present but usually there are no visible X-ray changes.

2nd stage arthritis Function of the joint is considerably disturbed, changes in the surrounding soft tissues are observable on X-ray and osteoporosis and subchondral sclerosis have begun.

3rd stage arthritis Function of the joint is greatly disturbed and there are advanced changes in the X-ray picture: osteophytes, degenerative cysts and other sclerotic changes in the epiphysis.

[3] Treatment with tetra-polar vacuum electrodes (Fig. 6.3) is mandatory in knee arthritis.

[4] Surgical treatment, and especially arthroplasty, has won recognition in treating arthritis of the hip. The application of pre- and postoperative kinesitherapy is of fundamental importance in such patients. As a rule, IT can be applied locally, but we prefer to act upon the segmental area. Interferential therapy is also recommended in treating all patients with hip arthritis in whom surgical treatment cannot be applied for one reason or another.

[5] In order to assess immediately the effect of IC and that of other physical methods in 60 patients with arthritis of the two knee joints, treatment was carried out with US, microwaves or diadynamic current on the left-hand side and with IC only on the right-hand side. As a rule IT was prescribed for the more affected joint. The effect in 14 of the patients was the same, but in 46 patients the effect was greater in the knee which received IC.

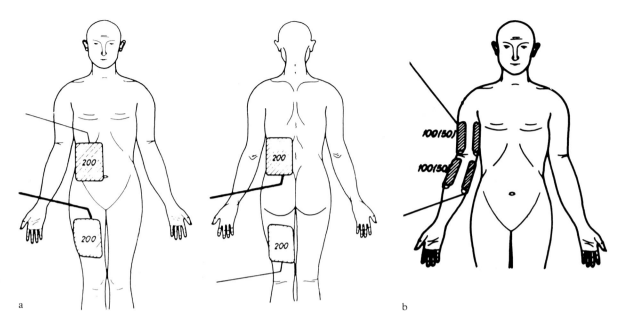

Fig. 6.1 Position of electrodes. a. Arthritis of the hip. b. Arthritis of the elbow joint.

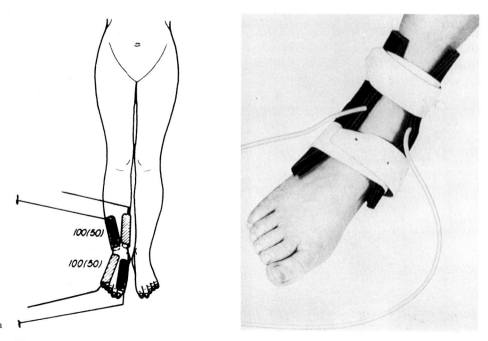

Fig. 6.2 Position of electrodes in treating knee joint arthritis. a. With 4-plate electrode. b. With 4-field electrode.

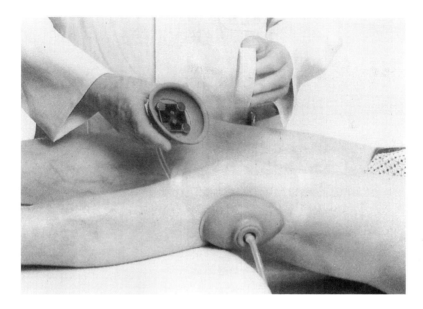

Fig. 6.3 Treatment of knee joint arthritis with tetrapolar vacuum electrodes.

apy too, the parallel or consecutive application of different methods being recommended. Jung & Gierlich (1968), for example, developed a method of combined application of diadynamic current and ultrasound (Sonodynator apparatus), and reported better results in various diseases of the locomotor system.

Since it was first introduced therapeutically, IC has been successfully combined with vacuum massage (e.g. Nemectrodyn apparatus) or infrared (Endogenos apparatus), but no studies have been carried out so far on its simultaneous application with other physical methods.

The lack of technical facilities at this stage for a simultaneous application of some physical agents (for example, ultrasound in an interferential current field) and the efforts to develop new, more effective methods, naturally led to the study of results with the application of two physical forms of treatment given consecutively. This is actually close to a simultaneous action, as both agents are applied without interval *immediately one after the other*.

In order to ensure more effective therapeutic combinations in knee joint arthritis, the effect of interferential current was studied by us first when applied simultaneously with ultrasound, then

Table 6.1 Sex and age distribution of patients with knee joint arthritis

Men	Women	21–40 years	41–60 years	61–75 years	Over 75 years
32(27%)	88(73%)	8	69	38	5

before ultrasound, and these two methods were compared with magnetotherapy, which has been recommended in the last few years.

Our observations included 120 patients with knee joint arthritis; their sex and age distribution are given in Table 6.1. The extent of the degenerative-dystrophic process is given in Table 6.2.

In the first group of patients (group I), IC and US were applied simultaneously,[6] while in the second (group II), US therapy was given immediately after interferential current. Ultrasound was applied using the labile technique at a dosage of 0.2–0.6 W/cm^2 over 8 to 12 minutes in 12 applications. Magnetotherapy (applied to group III patients) was conducted with an apparatus designed on the basis of technical data of the

[6] Ultrasound was applied in the area between the electrodes.

Table 6.2 Distribution of patients with knee joint arthritis by treatment groups and by extent of degenerative-dystrophic process

Extent of degenerative-dystrophic process	Number of patients		
	First therapeutic combination (Group I)	Second therapeutic combination (Group II)	Magnetotherapy (Group III)
0–I and 1st stage	18	17	17
I–II and 2nd stage	17	20	19
3rd stage	5	3	4

Soviet 'Polyus-1' apparatus. The knee joint was placed between the two inductors of the apparatus, the latter being closely applied to the skin. A continuous regime was used at a dosage of 25–40 mT for 15 minutes daily in 12, 15 or 20 applications. All the patients received out-patient treatment, without any drugs.

The therapeutic effect was assessed using the following indices: pain and function of the joint, X-rays, oscillography and rheography.

All patients under treatment complained of severe pain in the affected joints, especially at night and when descending and ascending stairs. Functional disorders were found in 85 patients

(27 from group I, 28 from group II and 30 from group III).

The following results were achieved in the three groups of patients: pain was favourably influenced (Fig. 6.4),[7] together with the muscular state and joint mobility (Fig. 6.5). The increased knee joint mobility is of great statistical significance ($p < 0.001$) for the three groups of patients.

Blood flow improvement in the area of the affected joint was demonstrated using oscillography and rheography in the three groups of

[7] Six of the patients (15%) treated with magnetotherapy were discharged without relief of pain.

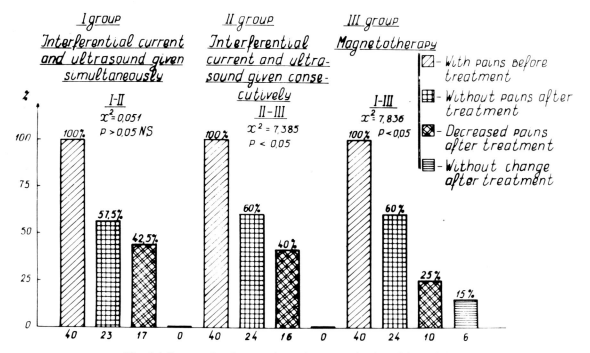

Fig. 6.4 Comparative therapeutic results on treating knee joint arthritis.

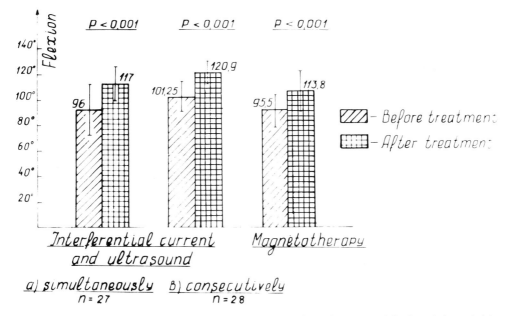

Fig. 6.5 Goniometric data on the function of the knee joint in patients treated for knee joint arthritis.

patients (Figs 6.6, 6.7 and 6.8). The control X-rays did not show any change in the X-ray appearance except in one woman from group I (periosteal reaction decrease in the metaphyseal area).

Results of treatment were followed up for 2 years, and all patients from group I and group II were reviewed. Recurrence (1–2 years after treatment) was found in 14 (35%) from group I and in 13 (32.5%) from group II, i.e. a lower percentage than in the isolated application of the two methods (Nikolova, 1973a). The ultimate results in 25 patients who benefited from magnetotherapy (group III) were reviewed within 20 days to 1 year after treatment. Relapse occurred in 4 (16%) after 1 month; in 6 patients (24%) after 2–6 months; in 6 (24%) after 9 months to 1 year—or a total relapse in 16 patients (64%).

These data show that:

1. Simultaneous or consecutive application of IT and US in knee joint arthritis helps give comparatively lasting relief of pain, with improvement or normalisation of the mobility of the joint. The clinical therapeutic result in both methods (i.e. simultaneous or consecutive) is equally effective. The immediate and later results are better than in the isolated application of the two agents. Preference should be given at present to consecutive application, as no adequate apparatus is available to enable safe application of US in the interferential current field.

2. Magnetotherapy has a beneficial clinical effect in the treatment of knee joint arthritis for a shorter length of time than does either IT on its own or IT used simultaneously or consecutively with ultrasound. Relapses are nearly twice as common and occur significantly earlier: in one study they occurred in the first 1–6 months in 10 patients (40%). Pain was also less influenced by magnetotherapy. Interferential therapy or its consecutive application with ultrasound are therefore preferable.

Spondylitic arthritis

Interferential therapy in the treatment of spondylitic arthritis has also given good results (Nikolova, 1971a, 1979). It is applied with 4-plate electrodes (or with 4 vacuum ones) positioned in such a way as to include the affected area of the

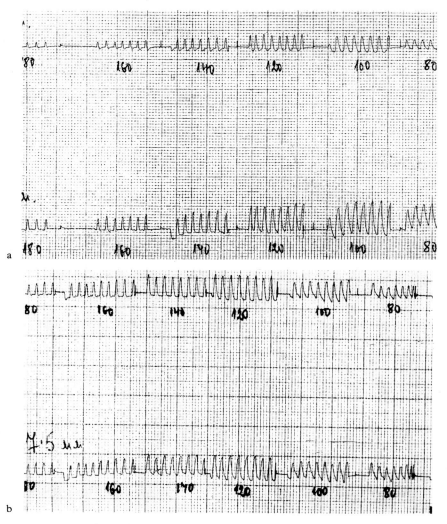

Fig. 6.6 Oscillography. a. Before treatment. b. After IT.

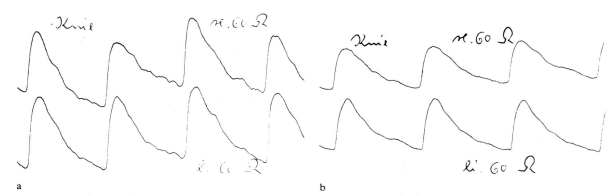

Fig. 6.7 Rheography of the left and right knee joints. a. Before treatment. b. After treatment with IC.

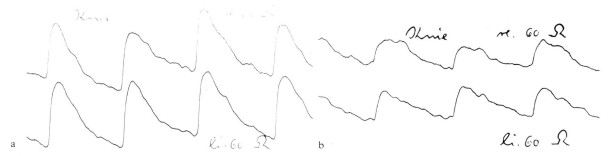

Fig. 6.8 Rheography of the left and right knee joints. a. Before treatment with IC and ultrasound consecutively — rheographic curve of angiodystonic type. b. After treatment — normal rheographic curve.

spine (Fig. 6.9). The bipolar electrodes are suitable (Fig. 6.10). A rhythmical frequency of 90–100 Hz is used in cervical arthritis, and in lesions of other areas a constant frequency of 100 Hz is applied in the first 3 treatments, and 0–100 Hz in the remaining ones. Treatment is given for 15 to 20 minutes, with a total of 20 per therapeutic course. Pain is usually relieved after the 5th treatment and disappears after the 15th to the 20th. Results are also beneficial in patients for whom other methods have failed. Repeated courses of treatment for persisting complaints are also effective. Very good results are obtained in combining IT with US and vacuum or manual massage.

Electro-acupuncture with IC gives very good results in treating cervical arthritis. Stimulation is given with a 4-point electrode (Nemectrodyn-8 apparatus) for 3 to 5 minutes on the following acupuncture points: GB 10, GB 12, GB 20, T 16, T 14, ST 15, BI 11, TH 15. A total of 10 treatments are carried out, and after a break of 8

to 10 days the treatment is repeated to strengthen the therapeutic effect.

Gouty arthritis was also favourably influenced by IT. The same method was applied as in osteoarthritis (p.60), and it was combined with adequate drug therapy to enhance the therapeutic effect.

Calcaneal exostosis

The treatment of calcaneal exostosis is both medical and surgical. Nearly all physiotherapeutic methods are used in medical treatment. Scientific publications on the effect of IC are scarce (Nikolova, 1971a; 1979). We started applying it as early as 1963, taking into consideration its pronounced pain-relieving effect and its regulating influence on tissue trophicity. A total of 80 patients have been observed. Complaints disappeared or were more or less reduced in 77 patients, and only 3 did not respond to treatment. Comparative studies on the effect of IC, micro-

Table 6.3 Results of various methods of treatment of calcaneal exostosis

Applied therapeutic method	Number of patients	Therapeutic results*			
		Healthy	Greatly improved	Improved	No improvement
IC	50	24(48%)	24(48%)	2(4%)	–
IC combined with microwaves	20	15(75%)	5(25%)	–	–
Microwaves	70	30(43%)	25(36%)	14(20%)	1(1%)
Ultrashort waves	25	3(12%)	15(60%)	6(24%)	1(4%)
Ultrasound	45	6(13%)	25(56%)	12(27%)	2(4%)

* Healthy = no pains or complaints. Greatly improved = substantial decrease of pain. Improved = minor decrease of pain

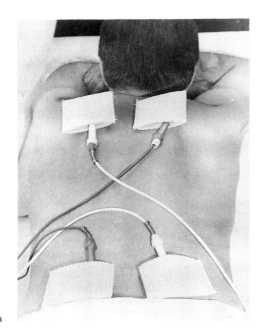

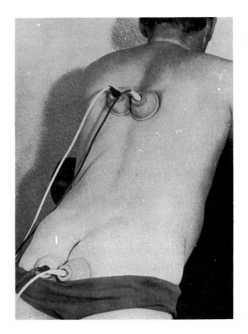

a

b

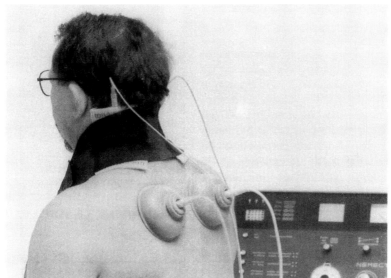

c

Fig. 6.9 Position of electrodes in treating spondylitic arthritis. a. With plate electrodes. b. With vacuum electrodes. c. Position of electrodes in treating cervical arthritis.

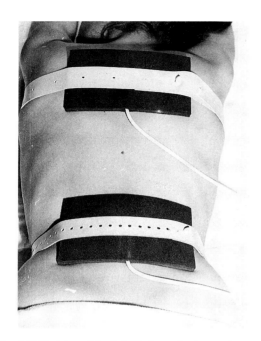

Fig. 6.10 Position of 2 × 2-field electrodes in treating spondylitic arthritis.

waves, ultrashort waves and US were carried out. The results are given in Table 6.3. They show that IT applied separately or in combination with microwaves gives the best results compared with the other physiotherapeutic methods.

Treatment is conducted with 4-plate or vacuum (in combination with vacuum massage) electrodes, or with the 4-field electrodes. The frequency of the current and the duration of the treatments are as in osteo-arthritis of the joints (pp.60–63).

7

Diseases and injuries of the nervous system

THE PERIPHERAL NERVOUS SYSTEM

Facial nerve palsy

Interferential therapy in the treatment of facial nerve palsy (due to cold, infection, injury) was introduced by us in this country in 1963 (Nikolova, 1966a). The analgesic effect of the current eliminates vascular spasm and stimulates the metabolic processes in the damaged nerve.

We observed and systematically followed up 170 patients. Their sex and age distribution are given in Table 7.1. The aetiological factors are presented in Table 7.2 and the duration of the disease in Table 7.3. As Table 7.3 shows, most patients were admitted for treatment after the 2nd month following the onset of the disease (a total of 99 patients or 58%).

The various medicines prescribed and the physiotherapeutic treatments carried out prior to admission had not proved effective. The clinical features were indicative of facial nerve palsy.

Interferential therapy (which cannot be applied any earlier than the 15th day following the onset of the disease) was carried out in the following two ways:

1. A 4-point electrode (T-white on Nemectrodyn-IV German apparatus) is placed as illustrated in Figure 7.1. Stimulation is applied with a rhythmical frequency of 0–140 Hz over a period of 8, 10 or 12 minutes.
2. The same method of stimulation is used over a period of 5 to 6 minutes and then

Table 7.1 Sex and age distribution of patients with facial nerve palsy

Men	Women	0–20 years	21–40 years	41–60 years	61–80 years
83	87	8	71	84	7

Table 7.2 Aetiological factors in patients with facial nerve palsy

Aetiology	Number of patients
Cold	34(20%)
Cold and infection	105(62%)
Otogenic neuritis	16(10%)
Trauma	9(5%)
Neuritis in hypertension	6(3%)

Table 7.3 Duration of facial nerve palsy at commencement of treatment

Duration of disease	Number of patients
Up to 30 days	31
31–60 days	40
61–90 days	39
4–6 months	27
6 months to 1 year	18
Over 1 year	15

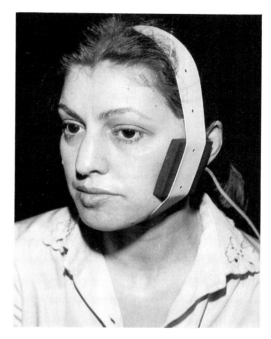

Fig. 7.1 Position of electrodes in treating facial nerve palsy (4-field electrode — small electrode in facial nerve palsy).

over a period of 3 minutes in the region of the oral and ocular angle of the affected side, but at a rhythmical frequency of 0–10 Hz, the aim being to produce muscle contraction.

A total of 12, 15 or 20 daily treatments are given.

In order to establish accurately the therapeutic benefit of interferential therapy, we used it on its own with no other additional therapy in 50 patients while in the other 120 patients IT was combined with ozocerite,[1] as it has been proved that the latter stimulates the regeneration of the

[1] Ozocerite is an oil product made in the USSR. 'Medical ozocerite' is used for medical purposes, water and mechanical mixtures having been removed from it. It has been found that, compared to therapeutic mud and paraffin, ozocerite possesses greater thermal heat capacity and the lowest heat conductivity. In addition, it contains biologically active substances with oestrogenic and acetylcholine-like effects. Ozocerite applications have been proved to stimulate regeneration processes in affected nerves.

affected nerve. The therapeutic effect was assessed on the basis of the clinical picture, routine electrodiagnosis and electromyography (EMG) (Fig. 7.2). Routine electrodiagnosis before and after treatment was carried out in all patients, and EMG in 40 of them (see Tables 7.4 and 7.5). The EMG examination data before treatment corresponded to results from routine electrodiagnosis, and after treatment improvement of EMG records was found in 17 patients before any changes were detected in routine electrodiagnostic (i.e. Faradic, galvanic) tests (see Glossary).

Following this treatment the clinical symptoms of the disease (i.e. inability to wrinkle the forehead, to close the eye — orbicularis oculi — etc.) completely disappeared in 38 patients, considerably decreased in 84 and improved in the remaining 48 patients (see Table 7.6). The positive effect was somewhat more pronounced in patients treated with IC and ozocerite applications, especially in those with severe partial denervation. The synergic action of these two factors can be assumed to lead to mutual enhancement of the therapeutic effects.

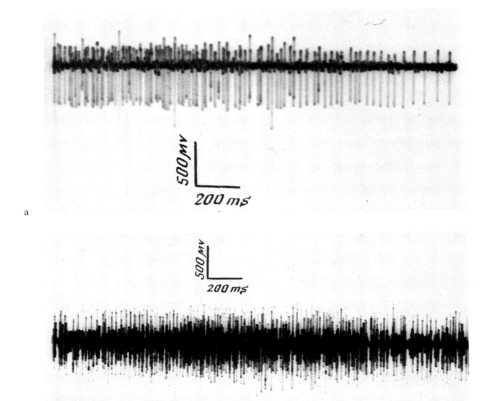

Fig. 7.2 Electromyogram in a patient with facial nerve palsy taken from orbicularis oris muscle. a. Before treatment — simple accelerated record. b. After treatment — greatly enriched record as compared to the initial EMG record.

Table 7.4   Changes following treatment for facial nerve palsy, as shown by electrodiagnosis

Routine electrodiagnosis	Before treatment	After treatment
Normal electroexcitability	–	7
Quantitatively decreased electroexcitability	4	7
Partial reaction of degeneration	146	139
Total reaction of degeneration	20	17

Table 7.5   Changes following treatment for facial nerve palsy, as shown by EMG

Electromyographic (EMG) changes	Before treatment	After treatment
Without EMG changes	–	4
Partial denervation:		
mild	20	24
severe	8	5
Total denervation	12	7

Our observations suggest that IC materially contributes to the functional recovery of patients with facial paralysis, the effect being less marked in severe lesions of the facial nerve. It should be further noted that in 3 of our patients with severe partial and total denervation, the decompression of the nerve was unsuccessful and subsequent treatment with IC resulted in substantial improvement in the patient's condition. This shows

Table 7.6 Results of IT treatment of facial nerve palsy

Applied therapeutic method	Number of patients	Therapeutic results[*]		
		Discharged healthy	Discharged greatly improved	Discharged improved
IC	50	11(22%)	24(48%)	15(30%)
IC and ozocerite applications	120	27(22.5%)	60(50%)	33(27.5%)

[*] 'Discharged healthy' = patients with restored function and without any complaints. 'Discharged greatly improved' = patients in whom the clinical symptoms of the condition have significantly subsided and electroexcitability has obviously improved. 'Improved' = patients with some clinical improvement, but without any change in electroexcitability. They were admitted with total or severe partial denervation, which is in line with Erb's concept that recovery in such patients is slow and problematic

that interferential therapy is important in the various stages of the evolution and treatment of facial palsy.

The effect of IT is illustrated by the following example:

A 28-year-old patient was admitted on January 31st, 1972 with a diagnosis of facial nerve neuritis (he fell ill on October 28th of the previous year). Data of partial reaction of degeneration were obtained by the routine electrodiagnostic method. The EMG of the orbicularis oculi muscle taken on February 2nd, 1972 showed single fibrillation potentials at rest; on moderate volitional contraction, bi-phasic and poly-phasic reinnervation potentials were shown with a duration of up to 3 msec and amplitude from 200 to 400 μV; on maximum volitional muscle contraction, an intermediate EMG pattern was shown with a time scale of 9.6 msec.

After interferential therapy the EMG showed lack of spontaneous activity at rest; on moderate contraction it showed polyphasic action potentials of a duration of 4 to 8 msec and amplitudes from 600 to 1800 μV; on maximum muscle contraction it showed a normal interference pattern with a time scale of 34 msec.

Serious therapeutic problems in facial nerve palsy include the pathological mass movements and contractures which occur usually as complications of severe involvement of the nerve and a faulty therapeutic approach. There is no uniform method of treatment of these rather unwelcome complications.[2] Interferential current at a constant frequency of 100 Hz was introduced by us in 1972/73 with a view to its sympathicolytic and beneficial action on tissue trophicity. Only the

[2] First of all, preventive measures are of the greatest importance in treating pathological mass movements and contractures. An adequate dosage of electrotherapy, massage and remedial exercises and electrical stimulation are applied only according to the electro-excitability tests.

region of the nerve trunk is stimulated at a dosage of 2–4 mA, so that the patient feels a slight but pleasant vibration. Sessions are provided daily for 6 to 10 minutes. After a few weeks' break the treatment can be repeated.

Twenty patients were treated using the method mentioned above, all of them with severe partial or total denervation. They benefited greatly from the therapy. The sensation of tightening in the affected facial area and the symptom of 'watering eye' decreased, as did the facial asymmetry at rest. The trick movements, i.e. the tic-like twitchings of the muscles, were also less common.

The treatment of secondary facial nerve palsy depends completely on the type and course of the basic disease. In paralysis of the facial nerve after removal of a neuroma in the cerebello-pontine angle, IC at a rhythmical frequency of 0–100 Hz gives a good result.

Occipital neuralgia

No data are available in the literature on the therapeutic effect of IC in treating occipital neuralgia. The treatment has been successfully applied by us in the following way: two 4-point electrodes are placed as illustrated in Figure 7.3. Current with a constant frequency of 100 Hz or a rhythmical frequency of 90–100 Hz is applied daily for 6 to 10 minutes for a total of 6 to 12 treatments.

Trigeminal neuralgia

Interferential therapy in the treatment of trigeminal neuralgia is applied with one 4-point (Fig.

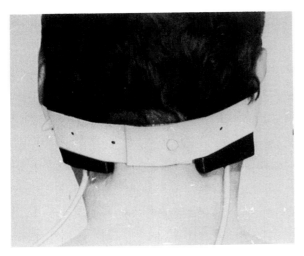

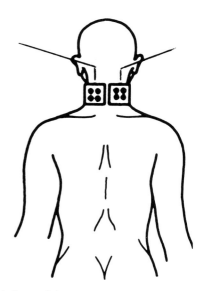

Fig. 7.3 Position of 2 × 4-field electrodes in treating occipital neuralgia.

7.4) or two 4-point electrodes (Fig. 7.5). A constant frequency of 100 Hz or a rhythmical frequency of 90–100 Hz is used. The first session lasts 5 minutes, and subsequent treatments for up to 10 to 12 minutes, when tolerance is good. A total of 6 to 12 sessions are recommended. In our experience the attacks occurred less frequently, decreased or completely disappeared.

Intercostal neuralgia

Interferential therapy in the treatment of intercostal neuralgia was first applied by Palairah et al

(1956). Four patients out of 5 recovered immediately after the first treatment, and 1 patient after the tenth. We have applied this method to 12 patients in whom pain disappeared after 10 to 14 treatments.

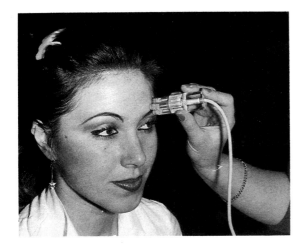

Fig. 7.4 Position of 4-point electrodes in treating trigeminal neuralgia.

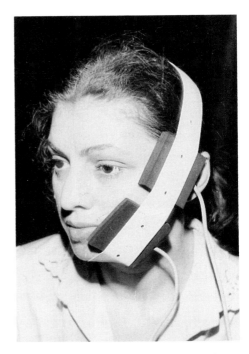

Fig. 7.5 Position of 2 × 4-field electrodes in treating trigeminal neuralgia.

The treatment is carried out with a 4-field electrode or 4-plate electrodes, positioned in such a way that the neuralgic region lies within the interference area of the two medium-frequency currents. A constant frequency of 100 Hz or a rhythmical frequency of 0–100 Hz is applied for 10 to 15 minutes daily, for a total of 15 treatments.

Brachial neuritis

Multiple therapy for conditions which involve the brachial plexus nerves includes a variety of physical agents with proven therapeutic effects. No clinical studies on the effect of IC are available in the literature. We have observed a total of 100 patients (60 women and 40 men), 92 of whom were aged between 20 and 60 years, and 8 patients over 60 years old. A traumatic aetiology was established in 4 patients; colds and infections accounted for the others. Together with the clinical examination, the patients were all X-rayed, and 51 patients had marked cervico-arthrotic changes. These data agree with the well-known fact that conditions causing brachial neuritis are often due to degenerative changes in the articulo-ligamentous mechanism of the vertebral column.

Previous treatment with drugs and physiotherapy (e.g. diadynamic current and ultratherm) had been given to 44 patients.

Interferential therapy has been carried out by us in the following way: 2-plate electrodes are positioned paravertebrally in the area of the lower cervical vertebrae, and the other two by the side of the wrist (Fig. 7.6). During the first 3 to 5 treatments a constant frequency of 100 Hz is applied followed by a rhythmical frequency of 0–100 Hz. Treatment is applied daily for 15 minutes for a total of 10 to 20 treatments.

The treatment of 10 patients was combined with massage and ozocerite applications; in 20 patients with cervical arthritis, treatment was combined with ultrasound applied paravertebrally. Remedial exercises were given to 25 patients after pain had been relieved.

All the patients were admitted in the acute or subacute stage with pronounced pain. The therapeutic results were assessed on the basis of clinical

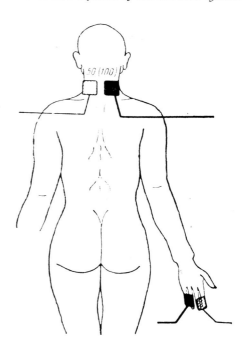

Fig. 7.6 Position of electrodes in treating brachial neuritis.

appearance, as well as oscillographic and electro-excitability investigations. A beneficial effect, including removal or reduction of the muscle wasting and trophic asymmetry, was found in all but 2 patients. Investigations showed, however, that complete functional restoration with IT is only achieved in 34% of patients, which suggests that in these cases IT would be more effective if applied as a component of a multiple therapy, particularly in cervical arthritis.

Interferential therapy is also effective in treating shoulder-hand syndrome. It is applied as in brachial neuritis, the shoulder joint being treated separately as well (Figs 7.6 and 7.7).

Lumbosacral plexus nerve conditions

Burghart (1951) applied IC in 341 patients with sciatica: healing was achieved in 84%, improvement in 7%, and the treatment was ineffective in 9%. The author has also carried out comparative studies on the effect of IT and other physiotherapeutic methods, such as ultrasound, ultratherm, microwaves, galvanic current and Novocain block. The data show that the best results were

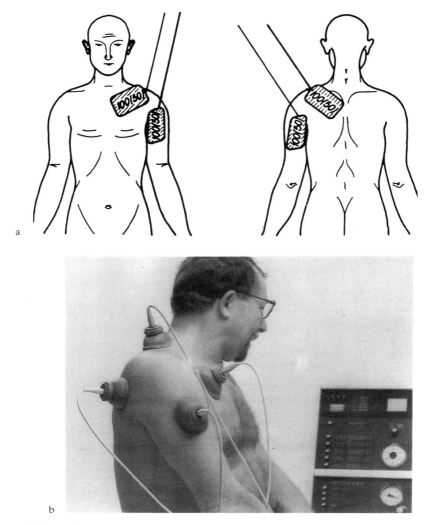

Fig. 7.7 Position of electrodes in treating disease of the shoulder joint (e.g. calcified bursitis and arthrosis). a. With plate electrodes. b. With vacuum electrodes.

achieved from interferential therapy. Thailhades (1959) achieved good results in treating toxic-infectious neuritis and radiculitis, as well as in 48% of the patients with sciatica.

We have applied IT in 100 patients with sciatica, aged between 22 and 70 years, using the following two methods of treatment:

1. Two-plate electrodes of an area of 200 cm² are placed paravertebrally in the lumbo-sacral region. The other two electrodes, 100 cm² each, are placed on both sides of the foot (Fig. 1.4). A current of a constant

frequency of 100 Hz or a rhythmical frequency of 90–100 Hz is applied for 10 to 15 minutes. As soon as the pain has disappeared, the rhythmical frequency is switched over to 0–100 Hz. In cases of lumbago the electrodes are placed in such a manner that the spinal muscles are in the region of the interferential field.[3]

2. Four electrodes are placed as follows: the first electrode is located paravertebrally in

---

[3] A combination of IT with vacuum massage is also recommended.

the L_3–L_5 region on the affected side, the second one over the ischial region, the third one on the common peroneal nerve around the fibula by the side of the popliteal fossa, and the fourth one on the inner edge of the foot (Fig. 7.8). One medium-frequency current is introduced through the first and third electrodes and another through the second and fourth electrodes. This method is suitable for overcoming pronounced pain and autonomic disorders. A constant frequency current of 100 Hz is applied. Pain is often relieved even after only 1 or 2 treatments.

The first method was applied in 56 patients with diminished and absent reflexes, muscle atrophy and sensory disorders, and the second method in 44 patients with pain manifested as sciatic scoliosis, muscle spasm and marked restriction of movements in the lumbosacral region. Interferential therapy was combined with infra-red in an additional 10 patients, and in a further 15 patients with discogenic sciatica, it was combined with traction therapy.

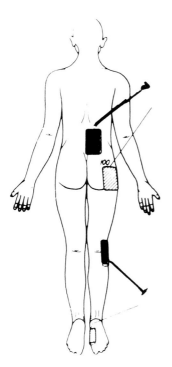

Fig. 7.8 Position of electrodes in treating sciatica.

In addition to the neurological pain-provoking tests, reflexes, sensory tests, electro-excitability and X-ray examination, the oscillographic index and skin sensitivity to ultraviolet rays was investigated in 70 patients before and after treatment. The marked asymmetry disappeared or was reduced after IT, which is an objective index of improved vascular tone and nerve function.

The clinico-therapeutic result was evident from the disappearance of pain or its substantial relief, increased or completely recovered range of movements, recovery of sensory disorders and muscle atrophy and improvement or recovery of electro-excitability. Patients with discogenic sciatica also benefited from IT. Function was restored in 12 patients (30%), improved in 26 (65%), and failed to restore in only 2 patients (5%).

Causalgia

The beneficial results of IT in treating causalgia were first reported by Thailhades (1959) and Polster (1965). It was Thailhades who showed the positive effect in 95% of the patients (relief of pain after some treatments) and pointed out the effectiveness of the therapy in recurring causalgia.

A well-known fact is that the disease develops after superficial injuries and incomplete interruption of peripheral nerves rich in sympathetic fibres (e.g. median, tibial and ulnar nerves). Usually 5 to 10 days after the injury various parasthesiae develop, and later on acute burning pains in the distal areas of the limbs, with concomitant autonomic and trophic disorders. There is irritation of the sensory and sympathetic fibres in the trunk of the peripheral nerve.

Treatment is multiple, involving both medicinal and physiotherapeutic methods and, when necessary, surgical intervention. Physiotherapy aims to relieve pain, improve blood circulation (vasodilating effect) and tissue trophicity and accelerate the regenerative process. Because of the mechanism of its action, IT is strongly indicated. The four electrodes are placed in such a manner that the two medium-frequency currents cross in the area of the affected nerve. A constant frequency of 100 Hz or a rhythmical frequency of

90–100 Hz is applied for the required 20 to 25 treatments of 15 minutes' duration daily. A greater or lesser positive effect is observed in all patients.

Phantom pains

In amputation stump and phantom pains, IT is directed through the segmental area. Two electrodes are placed paravertebrally, and two others medially and laterally above the stump itself. A rhythmical frequency of 90–100 Hz is applied in segmental stimulation and also 0–100 Hz in the second form of stimulation, to improve tissue trophicity and strengthen muscles.

Polyneuritis

Physiotherapeutic methods have long been applied in the treatment of polyneuritis of different types (infectious, exogenous, toxic-allergic, endogenous toxic). Preference is given to one or other physiotherapeutic method depending on the aetiology or the stage of the condition. No data on the application and effect of IT are available in the literature.

We have successfully introduced this method in the treatment of exogenous toxic polyneuritis (Nikolova, 1971a). Histochemical investigations carried out later on showed that this current improved the metabolism of the affected tissues and stimulated blood circulation and regeneration in injuries of the peripheral nerves. It also has an analgesic effect. This led us to study the effect of IC in treating endogenous toxic polyneuritis for patients with chronic renal insufficiency (CRI) receiving haemodialysis.

It is a well-known fact that polyneuritis in CRI patients undergoing dialysis is an extremely difficult problem. No reports are available in the literature so far on the application of physiotherapy in such patients except single studies on the use of remedial exercises, electrophoresis and syncardial massage (see Glossary) (Nikolova, 1971a) in diabetic polyneuritis.

Our observations covered 40 patients with CRI (Table 7.7), 28 men and 12 women, aged between 20 and 70 years. All the patients were admitted with the following subjective complaints: pain,

Table 7.7 Type of disease causing CRI

Disease which caused CRI	Number of patients
Chronic pyelonephritis	29
Chronic glomerulonephritis	9
Endemic nephropathy	2

paraesthesia, heavy gait or inability to move without help. To assess the effect of IT, the following indices were used: reflexes and sensory tests, skin thermometry and oscillography, routine electrodiagnosis and electromyography.

The subjective complaints were favourably influenced — there was relief or reduction of pain and paraesthesia, improvement in muscular strength, gait and reflexes, reduction of sensory disorders, improvement of data from routine electrodiagnosis, as well as a rise in skin temperature and oscillographic index with a decrease in asymmetry. The control electromyographic (EMG) examination in 7 of the patients also showed a beneficial effect, which was manifested by an improved conductivity rate in the nerves.

The results of these observations justify recommending IT as a component of multiple therapy for the polyneuropathy of patients with CRI, as well as for exogenous polyneuritis.

Stimulation was given simultaneously on the two limbs (Fig. 1.4) at a rhythmical frequency of 0–100 Hz for 15 to 30 minutes daily, with 25 treatments in total. Constant control and careful dosage of current intensity are required because of the sensory disturbances in the distal area of the limbs. Better results are gained when additional paravertebral stimulation is provided, the electrodes being placed in such a manner as to ensure crossing of the two medium-frequency currents in the area of the kidneys (a constant frequency of 100 Hz is applied for 15 minutes daily, for a total of 25 applications).

Peripheral nerve injuries

Increased automation and mechanisation of production processes and the constantly increasing number of traffic accidents have resulted in a growing number of injuries which affect the peripheral nervous system. Sometimes they are accompanied by other severe lesions such as fractures of bone. Treatment of peripheral nerve injuries is still a complicated and difficult task, all authors being unanimous in their opinion that it should be multiple and systematic.

The main problem both in the past and nowadays is to determine the position and severity of the injury and the indications for operation. Most patients are young or middle-aged. The hand nerves are most frequently affected (Herzog & Wilchelm, 1973).

Physiotherapeutic methods are widely used nowadays in the treatment and rehabilitation of patients with peripheral nerve injuries. They help to overcome shock ischaemia and functional block, prevent scars and adhesions, maintain the properties of muscle and ensure a better and faster recovery of function. The following methods have been tested and recommended at different stages of the therapeutic programme: electrical stimulation (Gutmann, 1958), massage and remedial exercises, electrophoresis with different drugs (galantamine hydrobromide, hyaluronidase, bendazol hydrochloride, etc.), US or phonophoresis, thermotherapy, hydrogen sulphide and radon tubs and occupational therapy (Mezzana, 1975).

Interferential therapy in the treatment of peripheral nerve injuries has been used by us since 1963; a rhythmical frequency of 0–100 Hz fulfils the basic therapeutic need. Based on clinical data, oscillography and classical electrodiagnosis (Nikolova, 1971a) we were able to show that the effect of IT was better than electrophoresis. Later, on the basis of the experimental data we obtained (Nikolova & Davidov, 1978) which testified to the stimulating effect of IC on regeneration processes, we continued our investigations. We focused our attention on electromyographic changes, whose diagnostic and prognostic significance has been pointed out by many authors.

Our observations covered a total of 105 patients with an age and sex distribution as shown in Table 7.8. The aetiological factors are shown in Table 7.9, and the nerves involved in Table 7.10. From Table 7.9 it can be seen that the greatest number of peripheral nerve injuries were produced by fractures (43%) and other limb injuries,

Table 7.8 Sex and age distribution of patients with peripheral nerve injuries

Men	Women	0–20 years	21–40 years	41–60 years	Over 60 years
64	41	21	45	33	6

Table 7.9 Aetiological factors in patients with peripheral nerve injuries

Aetiology	Number of patients
Fractures	45
Other injuries (traction of nerves, dislocation)	25
Pressure and overextension during operation	14
Obstetrical paralyses	5
Incised wounds	15
Gunshot wounds	1

Table 7.10 Patients with peripheral nerve injuries – nerve involvement

Involved nerves	Number of patients
Brachial plexus	27
Ulnar nerve	23
Radial nerve	19
Ulnar and radial nerves	7
Ulnar and median nerves	4
Common peroneal nerve	13
Common peroneal and anterior tibial nerves	1
Anterior tibial nerve	4
Other peripheral nerves	7

with a significant predominance of nerve involvement in the hand (Table 7.10).

The traumatic injuries of peripheral nerves were accompanied by the following complications: Sudeck's atrophy and delayed callus formation in 15 patients, myositis ossificans in 2, and elbow joint contracture in 11 patients. Surgical treatment was applied in 11 patients; neurorrhaphy in 5 and neurolysis in 6 patients.

The period from the injury to admission for treatment with IC is given in Table 7.11. It is evident that the majority of patients (55 in all) were admitted comparatively late — after the fourth month — and 22 patients (21%) were admitted too late — 1 to 10 years after the injury. Seventy-five patients had previous treatment with

Table 7.11 Length of time between injury and IT in patients with peripheral nerve injuries

Start of IT after injury	Number of patients
1 month	7
2 months	23
3 months	20
4–5 months	26
6–12 months	7
1–3 years	12
5–10 years	10

drugs and physiotherapeutic methods such as electrical stimulation, electrophoresis, mud applications and hydrogen sulphide tubs.

As was noted earlier, the purpose of physical therapy, as well as other kinds of treatment, is to ensure optimal conditions for nerve regeneration by relieving pain, maintaining muscle tone, preventing scar tissue formation, enabling its resorption, preventing contractures and deformities, and helping to disperse haematomata and to improve blood circulation. The mechanism of action of IC meets these requirements (Nikolova & Davidov, 1979).

Interferential therapy was applied at a rhythmical frequency of 0–100 Hz. The electrodes were placed in such a manner that the affected nerve was in the interference area of the two medium-frequency currents. Treatment sessions were conducted daily for 15 to 20 minutes, with a total of 25 in a therapeutic course. Interferential therapy was combined with remedial exercises or manual massage of the affected limb, and in 10 patients with ozocerite applications as well.

The therapeutic results were assessed on the basis of the following indices: neurological condition, oscillography, skin temperature tests, skin thermometry, routine electrodiagnosis and electromyography.

Table 7.12 presents the results. Routine electrodiagnosis and electromyography showed distinct improvement (Table 7.13 and Fig. 7.9). The 14 patients discharged with no change whatever in their condition after treatment had sustained severe intra-articular fractures: 5 had malalignment and elbow contracture; 4 had a long history of total denervation before and after treatment (over 4 to 10 years from the day of the injury); 3 had indications for surgical treatment (neurolysis); and there were 2 patients who subsequently benefited from postoperative IT.

Forty-one patients showed symmetrical oscillo-

Table 7.13 Electromyographic (EMG) changes following IT in patients with peripheral nerve injuries

Electromyographic changes	Before treatment	After treatment
Without EMG changes	–	6
Partial denervation:		
slight	15	27
severe	25	13
Total denervation	10	4

Table 7.12 Results of IT treatment of peripheral nerve injuries

Applied therapeutic method	Number of patients	Therapeutic results*		
		Restoration of function	Different degree of improvement	No change
IC combined with remedial exercises	54	26(48%)	22(41%)	6(11%)
IC combined with remedial exercises and ozocerite applications	10	4(40%)	6(60%)	–
IC combined with therapeutic massage	41	11(27%)	22(54%)	8(19%)

* 'Restoration of function' = healthy (no pain, clinical symptoms gone). 'Different degree of improvement' = relief or considerable reduction of pain and muscle atrophy, improvement of neurological condition, positive changes in routine electrodiagnosis and electromyography

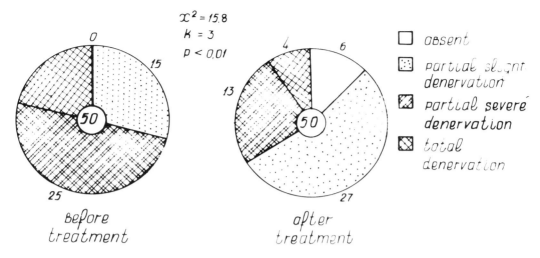

$x^2 = 15.8$
$k = 3$
$p < 0.01$

0
15
50
25

Before
treatment

4   6
13
50
27

after
treatment

☐ *absent*

⬚ *partial slight*
denervation

▨ *partial severe*
denervation

▧ *total*
denervation

Fig. 7.9 Electromyographic changes in peripheral nerve injuries before and after IT.

graphic indices and skin temperature tests, and a further 50 showed reduced asymmetry. This is indicative of the regulating effect of IT on vascular tone and blood supply in the affected limb. This fact is of great importance, as inadequate blood circulation can result in irreversible changes in the affected nerves (Gutmann, 1958). Both improvement of blood supply and relief of pain, along with preservation of muscle properties, are considered to be of the utmost importance in the treatment of peripheral nerve injuries.

EMG examination data before and after treatment in 50 patients suggest that IC stimulates the regenerative process mainly due to the improved and normalised metabolic processes, according to the evidence of appropriate histochemical examinations. Improved metabolism in the denervated muscular tissue after interferential therapy is particularly important and, if started early, no muscular atrophy develops. The fact that IT can disperse scars, adhesions and haematomata is also very important (Nikolova, 1971a; 1979). A decompression is produced, which enables the release of part of the blocked motor units.

The data obtained suggest that IT has a more pronounced effect when it is applied early in the first months after injury and when the injury is mild (partial denervation). Repeated therapeutic courses are required in other cases.

The importance of early treatment is stressed by most authors, but another fact should also be

borne in mind, namely, that the results of surgical treatment largely depend on pre-operative medication and rehabilitation procedures in the postoperative period, when prevention of postoper-

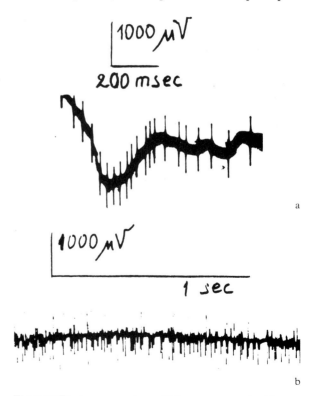

1000 μV
200 msec

a

1000 μV
1 sec

b

Fig. 7.10 Electromyography. a. Before treatment. b. After treatment — the EMG record is enriched.

ative scars is of the utmost importance for the final results. At this stage IT is particularly beneficial, all the more so if it can be started immediately, i.e. the day after the operation.

The effect of IT is illustrated by the following examples:

A 26-year-old patient was admitted for treatment with IC with a diagnosis of post-thyroidectomy and excision of lymphatic nodules — traumatic lesion of the axillary nerve.

Electromyography of the musculature innervated by the axillary nerve showed a considerably reduced number

of active motor units, severe partial denervation of the muscles explored, a simple EMG record and conduction velocity along the axillary nerve of 12 m/sec.

After IT and massage of the shoulder girdle for a total of 40 treatments, electromyography showed considerable improvement: the EMG record was enriched (Fig. 7.10a,b), and the conduction velocity along the axillary nerve was 33 msec; function was restored (Fig. 7.11a-f).

An 8-year-old patient sustained a supracondylar fracture of the right hand on September 10th, 1974. X-ray examination revealed a fracture with fragments displaced. Traction was applied for 15 days, followed by repeated reduction under general anaesthesia. The patient could not move the fingers of the right hand, which were numb, and had a lesion of the ulnar and median nerves. He was

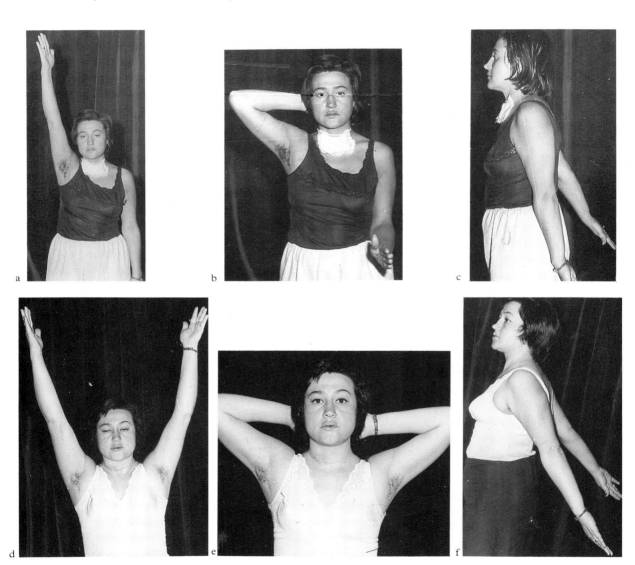

Fig. 7.11 Condition of the patient. a,b,c. Before treatment. d,e,f. After IT — functional repair.

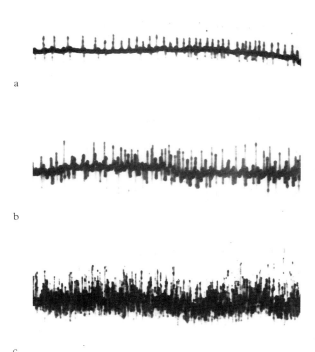

a

b

c

Fig. 7.12 Electromyography. a. Before IC treatment — simple EMG recording. b. After neurolysis but before IT — intermediate EMG recording. c. After IT — a rich intermediate to interfering EMG recording.

treated with galantamine hydrobromide tablets, vitamins B_1, B_6, B_{12}, and electrophoresis combined with galantamine hydrobromide, — massage and ultratherm — all unsuccessfully. The patient was admitted to hospital on November 2nd with a diagnosis of malunion of a supracondylar fracture of the right humerus, flexion contracture of right elbow, and traumatic lesions of the right median and ulnar nerves.

The EMG examination showed severe partial denervation of the abductor digiti minimi and dorsal interossei muscles (Fig. 7.12a) and total denervation of the abductor pollicis brevis muscle.

A total of 40 treatments with IC were applied. The elbow contracture was favourably influenced. As the control EMG did not show any improvement compared to the examination before treatment, a check-up was carried out and neurolysis of the ulnar and median nerves was performed. The neurolysis ensured partial improvement of motor unit activity (Fig. 7.12b), and after 20 treatments with IC, the EMG examination showed advanced reinnervation of the muscles supplied by the ulnar and median nerves (Fig. 7.12c). The patient was discharged with restored function (Fig. 7.13a–f).

Interferential therapy in the treatment of peripheral nerve injuries, as shown by our clinical

and experimental studies (see Part I), is a valuable therapeutic method which helps to relieve pain and vasodystrophic syndrome, to prevent muscle atrophy and to stimulate reinnervation. Early treatment ensures the best results, but IT is also effective in the later stages as well because of its general beneficial effect on tissue trophicity.

THE CENTRAL NERVOUS SYSTEM

Arachnoiditis

Surgical treatment is often the only effective method in spinal arachnoiditis, but postoperative systematic physiotherapy is also required. Interferential current helps to relieve or reduce both pain and adhesions. The therapy is the same as in spondylitic arthritis, combined with massage and remedial exercises. Also, in mild paresis the current is applied along the corresponding nerves at a rhythmical frequency of 90–100 Hz. In spastic paretic conditions the same frequency is used but at a low dosage.

Guillain-Barré syndrome (acute polyradiculo-neuropathy)

Interferential therapy is applied in residual phenomena in the affected area of the spinal cord (see arachnoiditis). Concomitant pelvic disorders are treated using the same methods as for nocturnal enuresis.

Myelitis

Physiotherapy is used in primary and secondary myelitis only as an accessory form of treatment. Some methods help to prevent complications such as pressure sores and contractures and to improve or restore motor function.

Interferential therapy is used in the chronic stage in the affected area (paravertebral positioning of the electrodes) at a constant frequency of 100 Hz and a rhythmical frequency of 0–100 Hz for 10 minutes daily, with 20 to 25 treatments in a therapeutic course. In slight paralysis the limbs involved are also treated (attention should be paid to sensory disorders). In spastic paresis and paralysis only a rhythmical frequency of 90–100 Hz is applied at a small dosage.

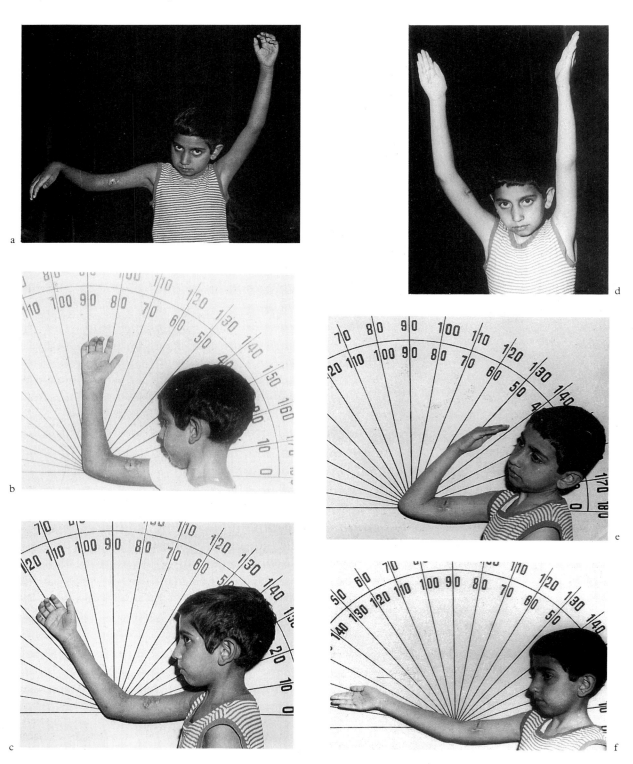

Fig. 7.13 Repair of function. a,b,c. Before treatment. d,e,f. After IC treatment.

Neurobrucellosis

Interferential therapy is also successfully applied in brucellosis lesions of the nervous system at a rhythmical frequency of 0–100 Hz. The position of the electrodes depends on the type of lesion. The duration of the necessary 15 to 20 treatments is 15 to 20 minutes. A combination of IT with thermotherapy (mud pack applications around the part), hydrogen sulphide or radon[4] baths is recommended.

Poliomyelitis

Interferential therapy in treating poliomyelitis was first applied by Nikoloff (1955), and later on by other workers, who established its beneficial effect in bringing about relief of pain, improvement of peripheral blood circulation and restoration or improvement of movement. It is used in the rehabilitation period and in the stage of residual symptoms. We applied this method in 20 patients, all of whom were in the residual stage and 8 of them had been affected for 3 to 10 years. A greater or lesser beneficial effect was objectively established in all of them by means of oscillography, rheography and electromyography. The aim of treatment was to act upon the spinal cord (Fig. 6.10) and the affected limbs. A constant frequency of 100 Hz was used to remove the autonomic disorders, a rhythmical frequency of 0–100 Hz to improve the trophic changes and to stimulate the regenerative processes and a lower rhythmical frequency for electrical stimulation. A total of 40 to 50 daily treatments were conducted for 15 to 20 minutes. A combination of IT with massage, thermotherapy or hydrotherapy is recommended.

Injuries of the brain and spinal cord

Interferential therapy in treating residual brain and spinal cord damage was first recommended by Thailhades (1959), who pointed out that it helps to restore functional activity. The electrodes are positioned according to the clinical symptoms. For instance, in spastic paraplegia the relevant segmental area is treated paravertebrally using a constant frequency of 100 Hz. Treatment relies on the antispasmodic action of this current to improve tissue trophicity. In atonic (flaccid) paraplegia both the affected segments and the limbs are treated. A current of a rhythmical frequency of 0–100 Hz is applied to improve the trophic changes and to strengthen the muscles. A total of 20 to 30 daily treatments or more are required for 15 to 20 minutes. Care is needed in selecting the dosage because of sensory disturbances.

THE AUTONOMIC NERVOUS SYSTEM

Acroparaesthesia

Acroparaesthesia, a paroxysmally occurring paraesthesia in the distal parts of the limbs, is a polyaetiological disease. It is often observed in women at the menopause, in cases of overfatigue, with frostbite and in other conditions. Treatment is both medical and physiotherapeutic. Interferential therapy gives very good results, the wrists being treated (Fig. 7.14), or the whole forearm, with plate electrodes at rhythmical frequency of 0–100 Hz, 10 to 15 minutes daily, for a total of 10 to 15 treatments.

Migraine

Interferential therapy in the treatment of migraine was introduced by Chappellart (1956), and later on some other authors pointed out its beneficial effect. Chappellart treated 20 patients distributed into 3 groups:

— group 1: Typical migraine syndrome with aura, unilateral headache, photophobia
— group 2: Migraine with concomitant liver disorders
— group 3: Migraine related to endocrine disturbances

The C_8–T_6 zone, the liver or solar plexus area were treated 3 times weekly for 20 to 30 minutes; a total of 6 to 12 treatments were given. Immediate results were disappearance of crises, later attacks becoming less frequent and of lesser intensity. The patients' sleep improved and

---

[4] Radon is a colourless, gaseous, radioactive element.

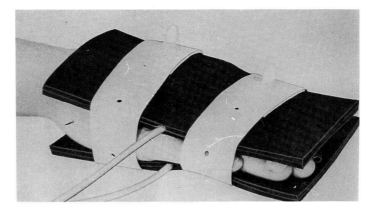

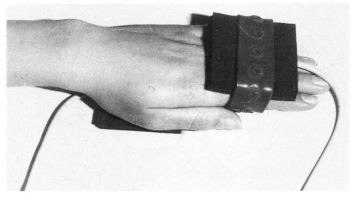

Fig. 7.14 Position of electrodes in treating acroparaesthesia.

diuresis increased. The author reports failure in 3 patients only.

The observations testify to very good results when IT is applied in the vasospastic form of migraine using the following method: a 4-point electrode (for superficial action) is positioned successively on the point of exit of the occipital nerve, on the temporal area and above the orbit. A current of a constant frequency of 100 Hz or a rhythmical frequency of 90–100 Hz is applied, the IT treatments being of 5, 10 and 12 minutes' duration, with 10 treatments constituting a therapeutic course. Electro-puncture by IC had also been successfully applied.

'*Vibration disease*'

Occupational dyskinesia (occupational coordination neuroses)

Tenosynovitis

8

Occupational diseases

'VIBRATION DISEASE'

During the past few years 'vibration disease' has come to the fore among registered occupational diseases and has acquired social significance. It has developed as a result of the continuous action of low- and high-frequency vibrations (240, 8000, 20 000 and 50 000 per minute) on workers under modern labour conditions in industry and agriculture. Vibration disease can be induced locally or generally. Two basic forms are differentiated at present, depending on the contact with vibrations:

1. Vibration disease due to local vibrations. This is observed in people working with manual vibrating instruments, machines and equipment. It is the classical form of vibration disease.
2. Vibration disease due to general vibrations.

The clinical picture of vibration disease is typified by four basic symptoms:

— neurotrophic (e.g. pains and sensory disturbances mainly of distal character)
— vaso-dystonic (e.g. angiospastic attacks, Palle's test[1] and spastic-atonic capillary network)

[1] Palle's test or test of the 'white spot': The researcher makes a digital compression on the dorsal surface of the patient's hand for 5 seconds, causing a white spot to appear on the compression area. The time necessary for restoration of the normal colour of the skin is measured. The normal restoration time is up to 5 seconds. More than 5 seconds is considered prolonged and is an indication of autonomic dystonia with sympathicotonia.

— osteo-articular and muscular (aseptic necroses, styloiditis, bursitis and other symptoms)
— auditory

These syndromes combine in different ways.

The evolution of the disease has four stages: *1st stage* — subjective complaints, mainly of paraesthesia and intermittent pains; *2nd stage* — moderate manifestations of the basic symptoms of the disease (e.g. paraesthesia, pain, angiospastic attacks, sensory disturbances), although the changes are reversible; *3rd stage* — trophic and degenerative alterations of the muscle, bone, tendon and articular mechanisms and metabolic disorders; *4th stage* — generalised lesions (e.g. sensory, trophic, cardiovascular), the changes being lasting and irreversible.

Vibration disease caused by general vibrations is different in form from the classical one, as its manifestations are dependent on the vibration frequency. The manifestations caused by high-frequency vibration are polymorphous, but disorders of the central nervous system are predominant. Signs of autonomic polyneuropathy are also found under the combined influence of general and local vibrations. Typical of low-frequency intensive vibrations are changes in the internal organs, the vestibular apparatus and bone.

The problem of treating vibration disease has attracted the attention of a number of specialists, and although much time has been devoted to it during the past few years, the problem has not yet been solved. Together with medical treatment (e.g. somniferous drugs, ganglion blockers, sympatheticolytic drugs, vitamins) a number of therapeutic methods including diadynamic current, ultrasound and microwaves are also being used for prophylaxis and rehabilitation.[2] The best results are considered to be obtained when medical treatment is combined with appropriate physiotherapy and the patient's work is interrupted. The purpose is to relieve the complaints and trophic disorders, restore disturbed function as much as possible and allow general strengthening of the body.

Interferential therapy in treating vibration

disease was first applied by us in 1969/70. The results in 25 patients observed during that period indicated a beneficial effect in 15 patients (60%) (Nikolova, 1971a). This encouraged us to continue our observations. A total of 60 patients, all of them miners, were systematically followed up. They were aged between 30 and 55, having worked with vibration instruments over periods of 5 to 22 years. Twenty-eight patients were in the 1st stage of vibration disease, and 32 patients in the 2nd stage.

Interferential therapy was applied at a constant frequency of 100 Hz simultaneously on the two hands: 2-plate electrodes were positioned paravertebrally ($C_3 - T_4$) in the cervico-thoracic area and two other electrodes were joined by a connecting cord on either side of the wrists. Fifteen to 20 daily treatments were performed for 12 to 15 minutes each.

The therapeutic results were assessed on the basis of the subjective complaints and the following indices: oscillography, skin thermometry, capillaroscopy, vibrosensitivity and the cold test with restoration of temperature.[3]

Table 8.1 shows that IT had a beneficial effect on all subjective complaints. Most pronounced was the therapeutic effect on general symptoms such as headache, vertigo, insomnia and heaviness

Table 8.1 The effect of IT on subjective complaints in patients with vibration disease

Subjective complaints	Before treatment	After treatment
Headache	43	11
Vertigo	41	7
Insomnia	48	12
Heaviness in heart region	31	3
Numbness of hands	55	29
Pain in hands	50	21
Whitening of fingers	43	10
Swelling of fingers	26	8
Hyperthydrosis	49	20

[2] There is no general agreement on their effect.

[3] The cold test with restoration of temperature: The skin temperature of the fourth fingertip of both hands is measured. The hands are immersed in water at a temperature of 4–5°C for 5 minutes. Then the skin temperature of the cooled hands is measured every 3 minutes until the temperature is restored to the initial level.

If the restoration of temperature lasts for 5 to 10 minutes and the temperature differences do not exceed 8 to 10°C, then the reaction is normal.

in the heart region. The best effect on local disorders was observed on vasomotor-trophic symptoms, and less marked on the subjective sensations of numbness and pain in the hands. Twenty-six of the patients had 'dead fingers' symptom before treatment and 11 after treatment, the attacks becoming less frequent and transient in all of them and affecting only the distal phalanges of the fingers.

The skin temperature before treatment showed considerably lower values (for the 4th finger and the forearm), and after treatment it rose by 1.16° to 3.4° — a statistically reliable change with a high level of significance ($p < 0.001$). However, the asymmetry of the skin temperature of the hands, which is characteristic of vibration disease, persisted after treatment.

Oscillographic recordings of the lower third of the forearm made before and after treatment showed that the oscillographic index was within normal limits in all patients, but asymmetry was found in 31. After treatment asymmetry was established in only 6 patients. In addition, after treatment, a tendency for reduction of the arterial tone and raising of the oscillographic index was noted in all patients. Statistical analysis did not show any significant difference ($p > 0.05$).

The capillaroscopic picture (of the 4th finger of both hands) has been followed up in 20 patients. Before treatment angiospastic anaemic syndrome with a pale yellow background was found in 12 patients with strongly constricted spastic capillaries and marked pericapillary oedema with opacity up to the apex of the capillary loops. Spastic-atonic capillaries were found in the remaining 8 patients. After treatment the capillaroscopic picture improved in 14 of the patients. In 10 of them it became almost normal, and in 6 it remained spastic-atonic. The positive changes in the capillaroscopic picture of the patients examined correspond to the raised number of positive capillaries for alkaline phosphatase observed experimentally (Nikolova & Davidov, 1979).

Vibrosensibility was measured in 20 patients by means of an electronic pallesthesiometer. Before treatment all of them showed reduced values and loss in decibels of various degree. After treatment vibrosensibility improved for low (50 Hz), medium (100 Hz) and high frequencies in both

hands of 14 of the patients — from 0.5 to 9.4 decibels. No changes were found in 3 of the patients, and in another 3 the threshold of vibrosensibility was raised.

The cold test with restoration of skin temperature (see footnote 3) was also performed in 20 patients. All of them showed abnormal initial values before treatment (25.3°–26.6°C) and prolonged recovery time. After treatment 13 patients showed normalisation of temperature values, of the reaction and the duration of recovery. The test did not show any change in 7 patients.

Skin temperature changes, the oscillographic index, the capillaroscopic picture, vibrosensibility and the cold test are all objective indices for measuring the regulating effect of IT on vascular tone. All these changes give grounds to consider IT as pathogenic in vibration disease. This is also confirmed by the positive effect of the current on the clinical symptoms of the disease.

Diadynamic current (diphasé fixe and short period modulation of 3 minutes), with paravertebral positioning of the electrodes at C_3–T_4, was applied in 20 patients, for a total of 12 treatments. When the effect of interferential current was compared with that of diadynamic current, both methods were found to have almost the same effect on general complaints such as headache and insomnia. The same applied to objective indices but with IT the capillaroscopic condition became normal earlier and more markedly.

OCCUPATIONAL DYSKINESIA (OCCUPATIONAL COORDINATION NEUROSES)

The overstrain of a given muscle group in doing certain work plays a leading part in the aetiology of occupational coordination neuroses, the prototype of which is writer's cramp. No agreement has been reached so far concerning the pathogenesis of the disease. It is generally accepted that treatment (medical and physiotherapeutic) should be started after interrupting the work which led to the disease for 4 to 6 weeks.

Interferential therapy in occupational dyskinesia was introduced by us. It is applied using the same methods as for vibration disease and brachial neuritis (Fig. 7.6). In addition, a current of a constant frequency of 100 Hz is applied for 15 minutes daily, for a total of 15 treatments, stimulating the cervical region (Fig. 6.9). As a result of the treatment, the patients' complaints are reduced or completely relieved.

TENOSYNOVITIS

This condition can be provoked by various causes, but it develops most often as a result of overstrain of the kinetic chain brought on by certain types of work.

Treatment in crepitant and serous tenosynovitis includes first of all functional rest and temporary immobilisation. Physiotherapy (microwaves, ultratherm and ultrasound for example) is an additional but important therapeutic method. Interferential therapy was recommended by some authors (Polster, 1965) but without any clinical analysis and precise therapeutic method.

We started a study of the effect of interferential therapy in treating tenosynovitis as early as 1963 (Nikolova, 1971a). Two hundred patients were systematically followed up — 56 men (28%) and 144 women (72%), with the following age distribution: 7 patients up to 20 years, 158 aged from 21 to 50 and 35 from 51 to 60 years. A traumatic aetiology was found in 6 patients, and the others could be considered to have sustained occupational microtraumata related to their profession (Table 8.2). Crepitant tenosynovitis was observed in 86 patients, serous in 64, and chronic tenosynovitis in 50 patients.[4] One hundred and

Table 8.2 Occupation of patients with tenosynovitis

Occupation	Number of patients
Labourers (bookbinders, plasterers and others)	35
Technicians, turners and computer operators	51
Medical workers (dentists, chemists, nurses)	39
Dressmakers, tailors and knitters	36
Typists	24
Musicians	12
Sportsmen	3

[4] Interferential therapy is contraindicated in tenosynovitis of tuberculous aetiology.

Table 8.3 Previous management of patients with tenosynovitis

Previous management before IT	Number of patients
Not treated	55
Treated with plaster splint only	73
Treated with splint, microwaves or ultratherm, electrophoresis, diadynamic current, drugs	72

ninety-one patients had a lesion of the flexors and extensors of the hand, and 9 of the Achilles' tendon.

The patients' previous management is shown in Table 8.3. Those treated with plaster of Paris immobilisation only for an average period of 10 to 20 days came immediately after its removal. A concomitant Sudeck's atrophy was observed in 7 patients with the disease, epicondylitis due to trauma was observed in 3 others and pes planus arthritis of the ankle joint and hallux valgus was seen in 1 patient.

All the patients were admitted with oedema along the affected tendon, pain on movement and disturbed function.

Interferential therapy was carried out with 4-plate electrodes placed so as to act upon the whole limb (Fig. 7.6). In the initial stage IC is of a constant frequency of 100 Hz (for marked pain relief and to reduce trophic changes) applied daily for 15 minutes in 15 to 25 treatments. Our observations so far have shown that the sooner the treatment begins, the better are the results obtained. In the chronic stage it is more suitable to apply IC at a rhythmical frequency of 0–100 Hz.[5]

The results of treatment with IT are given in Table 8.4. Only 9 of the patients (4.5%) were discharged without any improvement. Patients in whom subjective complaints and objective symptoms disappeared and function was restored were discharged as 'healthy'. These were mainly patients with acute tenosynovitis who had attended the Clinic in the first few days of the onset of the condition. The patients discharged 'greatly improved' and 'improved' were those in whom the subjective and objective symptoms were more

[5] Results in chronic tenosynovitis are better if IT is combined with US or phonophoresis with hydrocortisone.

Table 8.4 Results of IT treatment of tenosynovitis

Duration of disease	Number of patients	Therapeutic results*			
		Healthy	Greatly improved	Improved	No effect
2–10 days	52	37(71%)	12(23%)	3(6%)	–
15–30 days	65	31(47%)	20(30%)	12(20%)	2(3%)
40–60 days	48	15(31%)	21(44%)	10(21%)	2(4%)
Over 4–6 months	20	4(20%)	6(30%)	7(35%)	3(15%)
Over 6–12 months	15	3(20%)	4(27%)	6(40%)	2(13%)

* 'Healthy' = function restored. 'Greatly improved' and 'Improved' = reduction in subjective and objective symptoms.

or less reduced. The lowest figure is the percentage of improvement in patients with the chronic form of the disease. It should be noted that in patients who benefited from IT, a reduction of asymmetry was found in the oscillographic index and skin sensitivity to ultraviolet rays, which is indicative on the one hand of disturbed vascular tension in tenosynovitis, and on the other of the regulating effect of this current on vascular tension.

If surgical treatment is required in chronic tenosynovitis, IT is provided postoperatively at a rhythmical frequency of 0–100 Hz as it helps to relieve pain and restore function.

9
Skin diseases

ACNE VULGARIS

Interferential therapy in treating acne vulgaris was first successfully applied by Meyer in 1953. He claims that a beneficial effect can be obtained even after 2 to 3 treatments. The affected area is stimulated with a 4-point electrode at a rhythmical frequency of 0–100 Hz for 20 minutes. The number of treatments is determined as required. Observations made by us coincide with those of Meyer.

HERPES ZOSTER

The positive effect of IT in treating herpes zoster was first proved by Meyer in 1952. It is confirmed both by other authors and by some of our observations.

So far we have applied IT in 25 patients, 10 men and 15 women. In age, 20 patients were up to 50 years and 5 were between 60 and 70. Three patients had residual neuralgia, and the others were admitted between the 5th and the 15th day after the onset of the disease. Intercostal herpes zoster was diagnosed in 19 patients, brachial in 6. Table 9.1 shows the results we obtained as well as comparing IT with other methods. As the table indicates, we obtained a therapeutic effect with IT similar to the effect of microwaves and considerably better than the effect of diadynamic current and ultraviolet erythematous irradiation. The treatment is conducted with 4-plate electrodes of an area of 50 or 100 cm^2 each, positioned

Table 9.1 Results of IT and other treatments of herpes zoster

Applied therapeutic method	Number of patients	Therapeutic results*		
		Healthy	Considerable improvement	Improvement
IC	25	18(72%)	7(28%)	–
IC combined with microwaves	5	5(100%)	–	–
Microwaves	20	17(85%)	2(10%)	1(5%)
Diadynamic current	20	4(20%)	14(70%)	2(10%)
Ultraviolet erythematous irradiations	12	4(33%)	6(50%)	2(17%)

* 'Healthy' = no complaints, no rash, without residual neuralgia. 'Considerable improvement' = subjective complaints and objective symptoms have almost disappeared. 'Improvement' = reduction of pain, rash, skin eruption

in such a manner that the crossing of the two medium-frequency currents should be in the affected area. A current of a constant frequency of 100 Hz or a rhythmical frequency of 90–100 Hz is applied. The necessary 6 to 15 treatments are provided daily over a period of 15 minutes each.

Interferential therapy can also be combined with vacuum massage in the treatment of herpes zoster.

PENILE INDURATION

This disease is characterised by fibrosclerous changes of the cavernous bodies of the penis causing distortion and functional disorder. The aetiology and pathogenesis of the disease have not yet been elucidated.

Ultrasound, phonophoresis with Aminosine (tiosinamine) ointments and potassium iodine (KI) electrophoresis have been successfully applied so far.

Interferential therapy in the treatment of penile induration was introduced by Meyer (1952). He obtained complete restoration of function in 7 out of 14 patients. The author recommends at least 20 treatments per therapeutic course. He also claims that ultrasound combined with IC gives much better results than when they are used separately. The reason he gives for this improved result is the enhanced dispersing effect of ultrasound on the fibrosclerotic changes, added to the analgesic effect of IC, which improves tissue trophicity.

Treatment was carried out with 4 small-plate electrodes 2–3 cm^2 each, positioned so that the

two medium-frequency currents crossed in the indurated area. A current of 0–100 Hz at a rhythmical frequency was applied. The treatments were given daily or every other day for 15 minutes for a total of 10 to 20 treatments. Pain disappeared, softening of the penis was observed, and erection and sexual intercourse became possible.

NEURODERMATITIS

Interferential therapy is suitable in mild strength for treating itchy patches caused by neurodermatitis. It is applied at a constant frequency of 100 Hz for 10 minutes to each patch, for a total of 15 to 20 treatments.

LESIONS DUE TO X-RAYS AND RADIUM RAYS

Interferential therapy for treating lesions due to X-rays or radium rays was applied for the first time by Meyer (1952) and Terrier (1954). Positive results were reported later by other authors as well (Polster, 1965). All authors stress that the results obtained are very good, even in long-term necroses and radiodermatitis where treatment by other methods has failed. But very often, more than 20 treatments are required.

Interferential therapy is applied with 4-plate electrodes placed so as to include the region of the ulcer in the interference zone. A current of a constant frequency of 100 Hz and a rhythmical frequency of 0–100 Hz is used. The procedures are carried out daily for 30 minutes, with 20 to 30 or more in a therapeutic course.

Interferential therapy gives convincing results in the treatment of sluggish wounds due to electric shock, as well as for indolent wounds.[1]

---

[1] Polster (1965) also recommends IT in treating psoriasis vulgaris. However, as we lack any personal experience in this area, we cannot give an assessment of the method. The therapy is also applied by others for cosmetic purposes, such as removing forehead wrinkles and double chins and for strengthening the facial muscles.

10

Surgical conditions

DISEASES OF ARTERIES AND VEINS

Buerger's disease (thrombo-angiitis obliterans)

Leo Buerger gave the classical description of this disease as early as 1898 but its aetiology and pathogenesis have not yet been fully clarified. Nowadays it is considered to be a general nervous-dystrophic disease affecting mainly the vascular system. Three forms of the disease are differentiated: angiospastic, thrombo-angiitic and angiosclerotic.

The evolution of the disease undergoes three stages: spastic, spastic-paretic and ulcerous-gangrenous. Basic therapeutic tasks are to remove all factors leading to peripheral vessel spasm; to remove the spasm itself; and to stimulate the collateral blood circulation. At certain frequencies IC has vasodilating and pain-relieving effects as well as improving tissue trophicity. For these reasons IC long ago attracted the attention of specialists with a view to its application in Buerger's disease. As early as 1953 Kaindl, Pärtan and Warum reported the positive effect of IC on the condition manifesting itself in reduced or relieved pain and trophic changes and an improved oscillographic index and rheograms, the patient being able to cover longer distances without pain.

Interferential therapy is given in three ways:

1. Using a ganglion cervico-thoracic block when the upper extremities are affected. The lumbar segmental area is acted upon in diseases of the lower limbs.

2. Using a sympathic trunk block at a constant frequency of 100 Hz.
3. Local action on the extremities involved. Four-plate electrodes of 100 cm^2 each are applied. Two of them are positioned paravertebrally at the 1st to the 3rd vertebral level and the other two on the distal part of the extremity. Simultaneous treatment of the two limbs can be carried out using six electrodes and a connecting cable (Fig. 1.4). A constant frequency of 100 Hz is applied in the first 3 treatments, and a rhythmical frequency of 0–100 Hz in the remainder for 15 to 25 minutes each. Altogether there are 15 to 30 treatments.

The first and second method can be used in all the three stages of the disease, and the third one in the first and second stage. Arterial spasm is easier to remove and collateral circulation is increased when the segmental action is alternated with a local one over the extremities affected, which is appropriate to the first and second stages of the disease.

Interferential therapy was applied in 90 patients — 89 men and 1 woman — with the angiosclerotic form of Buerger's disease. Fifty-seven patients were aged between 30 and 50 years, and 33 between 51 and 70. Thirty-four patients were in stage I, 52 in stage II, and 4 in stage III of the disease. All of them entered the Clinic after examination in the surgical clinics of the Medical Faculty in Sofia followed by medication, Novocain blocks or physiotherapy. Sympathectomy in 5 had failed.

After the first 12 IC treatments pain diminished and the extremities became warmer. Thirty-eight patients were discharged 'clinically healthy' (no subjective complaints, easy gait); 36 patients with 'great improvement' (essential decrease of subjective complaints, 5 times — or more — greater walking distance able to be covered daily without pain); 12 with 'improvement' (decrease in subjective complaints, 3 times greater walking distance without pain); and 4 patients did not benefit from the treatment.

The following results were found on completion of therapy:

1. Disappearance or reduction of trophic disorders in 86 patients, no change in 4.

2. Increase in the oscillographic index by 1 to 3 mm, on average.
3. Restoration of arterial pulses, which were weakened or absent before treatment, in 71 patients.
4. A rise in skin temperature in the treated extremities by 1° to 4°.
5. Shortening of the lengthened pulse wave time due to the disease and improvement in the pulse curve image in the oscilloscope of the Syncardon apparatus. This objective test is considered by many authors as more reliable in diagnostic and prognostic aspects than oscillography.[1]
6. Improvement in the rheographic curves taken in 20 patients (Fig. 10.1) before and after treatment.
7. Increase in the distance which the patient is able to cover without pain when walking from 250–400 m to 3–5 km or more.
8. A beneficial effect in patients for whom sympathectomy had failed. This is supposed to be due not only to the innate properties of IC but also to the fact that the current acts in an environment which has been favourably altered because of the operation.

Analysis of our results when using IT and other physiotherapeutic methods (Nikolova, 1970e) showed reduction or remittance of clinical symptoms and improvement of objective parameters when applied in the first and second stage of the disease. Periodic applications of interferential therapy (2 to 3 times annually) in the first and second stage maintains the patients and their capacity for work.

Physiotherapy in itself, whatever the method used, cannot solve the problem of how to treat Buerger's disease successfully, but it has proved very useful as a component of a multiple therapy when it is applied systematically and at the right time; a combined action between physical and other therapeutic methods is most desirable. On the whole, separate methods should not be

[1] Dimitrova (1977) found that the oxygen rise in venous blood above the norm in second stage patients falls after IC is applied, which is objectively indicative of improved collateral blood circulation after interferential therapy.

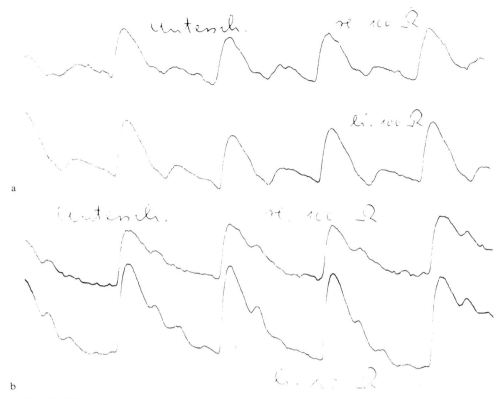

Fig. 10.1 Rheography in a patient with Buerger's disease. a. Before IT. Rheographic curves of angiodystonic type, the atonic manifestations prevailing; slightly lowered amplitude and rheographic index; slightly decreased angle of the anacrote; slightly lowered relative pulse volume and rheographic quotient; slightly lengthened time of the anacrote, a hardly rounded rheographic peak; secondary waves also outlined in the lower third of the anacrote. b. After IT. Normal amplitude of the rheographic index; normal angle of the anacrote; normal values of the relative pulse volume and rheographic quotient; normal time of the anacrote; normal and sharp rheographic peak; secondary waves are also outlined in the middle third of the anacrote.

opposed to each other, but should combine or alternate depending on the patient's condition. Treatment of patients with Buerger's disease must be conducted with the closest co-operation between the surgeon and the physiotherapist. Certain therapeutic agents can also be combined depending on the stage and form of the disease and the individual condition of each patient. For that reason physiotherapeutic regimes cannot be schematised. In our experience, the best results are achieved in patients in the first and second stage when IT is combined with syncardial massage and adequate chemotherapy, and when the different methods are alternated.

Since 1984 we have used electro-puncture with IC in treating patients with angiospastic and angiosclerotic forms of the disease. A rhythmical frequency of 0–10 Hz for 2 minutes is applied on the following acupuncture points: BI 25, BI 31, BI 33, BI 34, BI 49, GB 30, ST 36, LI 4, TH 5, BI 60, KI 3 and GB 39.

Raynaud's disease

Treatment of Raynaud's disease is both conservative (medical and physiotherapeutic) and surgical. The basic aim of each type of treatment is to regulate the vascular tone. It is agreed that physiotherapy has to be directed not only to local disorders but also to the relevant segments of the nervous system (general and reflex-segmental action). The vaso-motor and trophic disorders are related to the pathological state of the vascular centres.

Interferential therapy in the treatment of Raynaud's disease (Nikolova, 1971a, 1979) is applied in two ways:

1. The whole extremity is acted along, as in brachial neuritis (Fig. 7.6), at a constant frequency of 100 Hz. A total of 15 to 20 treatments are given daily for 10 to 15 minutes each.
2. A cervico-thoracic ganglion block is applied, using a 4-point electrode. Treatments are carried out 3 times a week for 10 minutes, with 10 in a therapeutic course.

The block is not recommended in patients susceptible to collapse and in those with an organic heart defect. For that reason we prefer the first method.

Interferential therapy proved to be suitable mainly in the first and second stage of the disease. It was applied in 40 systematically reviewed patients (7 male and 33 female), 35 of them aged between 20 and 40 years, and 5 between 41 and 55. The upper extremities were involved in all patients but 1. Fifteen patients were in the first stage of the disease and 25 in the second. The complaints had persisted for between 1 and 5 years. No data indicative of another disease were obtained from the clinical investigations. All the patients were subjected to preliminary treatment with vasodilating drugs, Novocain block or hydrotherapy.

To assess the effect of treatment, the following objective indices were used: oscillography, skin thermometry and skin sensitivity to ultraviolet rays (UVR) through defining the test dose in 35 patients. Asymmetry in the values of the given indices was found in 29 patients before treatment.

After treatment subjective complaints were eliminated and trophic changes were favourably influenced in 15 patients, having diminished to a different extent in the remaining 25 patients.[2] Control investigations of oscillographic index, skin temperature and skin reaction to UVR showed disappearance or levelling of asymmetry

in all patients with the exception of 1.[3] Patients discharged without complaints were reviewed within 6 months after treatment. Recurrence was found in 2. Repeated IT also yielded positive results and is therefore recommended 2 to 3 times a year.

Diabetic gangrene

Diabetic gangrene is treated either surgically or by drugs, IC being used only as an additional treatment, together with other physiotherapeutic methods, for instance microwaves and syncardial massage. Interferential current is successfully applied in the segmental area at a constant frequency of 100 Hz for 15 minutes daily, for a total of 20 to 25 treatments. Simultaneous action is produced along the affected extremity, the first 2-plate electrodes being positioned in the appropriate segmental area, and the other two above the area involved in the gangrene, on intact skin. A constant frequency of 100 Hz is applied for 10 minutes. A total of 25 treatments or more are needed. If necessary, treatment can be repeated after a 15-day break. Interferential therapy has been successfully applied in combination with syncardial massage, the procedures being alternated every day or every other day.

Varicose veins

Treatment of varicose veins is both medical and surgical. A number of physical methods such as long wave diathermy, syncardial massage, diadynamic current and some hydrotherapeutic procedures have been successfully applied, when used in the initial stage of the disease.

Interferential current was first applied by Burghart (1952) to stimulate venous flow and to improve vascular wall tension. Four-plate electrodes are placed so that the two medium-frequency currents cross in the varicose vein area (Fig. 10.2).[4] A rhythmical frequency of 0–100 Hz is applied up to the 4th treatment, and then 0–10

---

[2] The attacks became less common, of lesser intensity and with less marked trophic changes.

[3] These data are an objective index of the regulating effect of interferential current at a constant frequency of 100 Hz on the vascular tone in patients with Raynaud's disease.

[4] Treatment is also conducted with 2-field electrodes (Fig. 10.3) and vacuum electrodes.

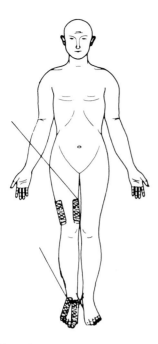

Fig. 10.2 Position of plate electrodes in treating varicose veins of the lower leg.

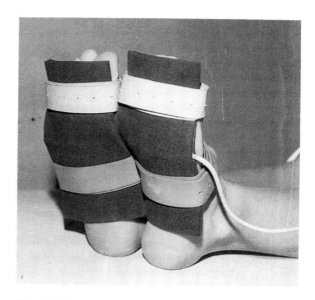

Fig. 10.3 Treatment of varicose veins with 2 × 2-field electrodes.

Hz daily for 15 to 20 minutes in the 20 required procedures.

Interferential therapy was applied by us in 80 patients with varicose veins in the initial stage. All of them benefited from the treatment: the pain subsided and the feeling of heaviness in the limbs and trophic disorders diminished, which can be explained by the improved tension of the venous walls. Comparative investigations on the influence of long wave diathermy, syncardial massage and diadynamic current (Fig. 10.4) showed that IT was the most effective treatment (Nikolova, 1971a, 1983). An essential advantage of interferential therapy is to maintain improvement, if applied periodically (2 to 3 times a year).

Interferential therapy is also effective in the treatment of varicose ulcers. The current is applied both on the ulcer[5] and over the whole extremity at a rhythmical frequency of 0–100 Hz for 10 to 15 minutes in 20 treatments. It is advisable to combine IT with US or syncardial massage, the treatments being alternated every

[5] The plate electrodes are positioned so that the ulcer is in the interference area of the two medium-frequency currents.

other day or carried out in sequence (Nikolova, 1970e, 1979).

SKIN CONDITIONS

Burns

Interferential therapy in the treatment of burns is recommended mainly in residual sequelae. It is carried out by means of 4-plate electrodes positioned so as to enable the crossing of the two medium-frequency currents in the burnt area. A constant frequency of 100 Hz and a rhythmical frequency of 0–100 Hz are used. The 20 treatments required are given daily for 15 to 20 minutes. Local lesions due to electric burns and lightning also respond well.

Frost bite

The beneficial effect of IT in treating frost bite was observed by Burghart (1951) and Terrier (1954). Interferential therapy can be applied in all stages of frost bite using a segmental technique. It is especially effective in sequelae to frost bite (e.g. pain, cyanosis, scars). In principle treatment is carried out as for thermal burns. Not less than 10

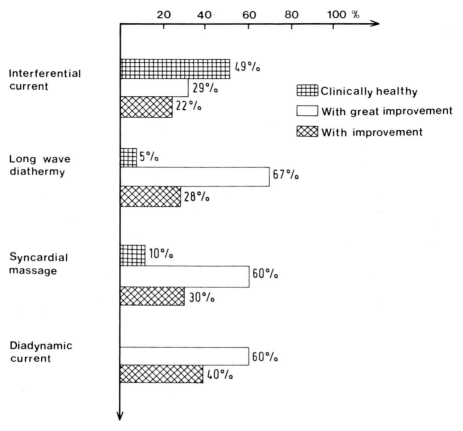

Fig. 10.4 Results of applied physiotherapeutic methods in treating varicose veins. 'Clinically healthy' = the patient's complaints disappeared (strain, feeling of heaviness in the limbs, exhaustion), the slight swelling around the ankle and dorsum pedis also disappeared, and there was considerable diminishing or disappearance of trophic disorders. 'With great improvement' = removal or considerable decrease of subjective complaints; significant improvement of objective changes. 'With improvement' = subjective complaints decreased, but without considerable improvement of trophic disorders.

to 15 treatments are recommended twice daily over a period of 15 to 30 minutes.

Chilblains

Interferential therapy for treating chilblains was introduced by us (Nikolova, 1971a). The 2-field electrodes are most suitable or 4-plate electrodes positioned so that the involved areas are in the interference zone. Out of the 12 to 20 treatments required, the first 3 are given at a rhythmical frequency of 90–100 Hz and the remainder at a frequency of 0–100 Hz for 10 to 15 minutes daily. Positive results are obtained essentially because of improved blood and lymphatic circulation.

LESIONS AND DISEASES OF BONE

Fractures*

The basic treatment for all types of fracture is surgical. However, physiotherapy plays an important part both in preventing complications and in aiding functional recovery.

Treatment of fractures aims at: (a) complete anatomical repair of the broken bone (reduction

---

* Professor Dr Georgi Balchev, an orthopaedic-traumatologist, for whose valuable collaboration we are greatly indebted, has been consulted about all patients cited in this and the following sections. The effect of interferential therapy has been estimated jointly.

and fixation) and (b) complete restoration of function. Adequate rehabilitation is as important as correct reduction.

Timely consolidation of the broken bones, prevention of complications, as well as complete restoration of function are best achieved when accurate reduction and immobilisation are combined with early and systematic application of adequate physiotherapeutic treatment. Therefore surgical and physiotherapeutic management must be combined and continued until complete restoration of function is reached. This requires a constant and close collaboration between the surgeon and the physiotherapist. When physiotherapy is prescribed, one has to consider the type of fracture, the stage of the condition, the effect of different physical methods, the time required for consolidation of the bones and the general condition of the patient.

There are some references in the literature which relate to the effect of IC on fractures (Wolf, 1956; Fiedler, 1960), but no data are available on the techniques and mechanism of stimulation of bone regeneration.

Treatment with IT has been used by us in fractures since 1963, and with a prophylactic purpose in recent fractures (i.e. still in the period of immobilisation) since 1966. The effect on the fracture is determined by the time of starting treatment and by the therapeutic purposes. Immediately after reduction and immobilisation, the surgeon is faced with pain, oedema and muscle spasm. We have tried to relieve pain and oedema, accelerate the absorption of haemorrhage and create conditions for a more rapid regeneration of bone tissue, i.e. to prevent complications. By the mechanism of its action interferential current completely meets these requirements.

Interferential therapy during immobilisation is conducted in the following way: apertures are cut out in the plaster for the 4-plate electrodes, or the electrodes are positioned in unplastered areas so that the two medium-frequency currents cross in the fracture area. It is also effective to encircle the whole extremity widely, or to place the first two electrodes paravertebrally in the relevant segmental area and the other two in the distal part of the affected limb. Treatments are given daily over a period of 15 to 20 minutes. Ten days after the

injury a rhythmical frequency of 0–100 Hz is applied because of its analgesic effect and its ability to normalise tissue trophicity. Then a constant frequency of 100 Hz is used, because of its spasmolytic and analgesic effect, to stimulate callus formation.

Our observations on 50 patients with different fractures showed that IT during immobilisation is a valuable preventive measure against complications after fractures, such as articular rigidity, muscle atrophy and retarded callus formation, and it also shortens the time of restoration of function after removal of fixation (Nikolova, 1971a, 1979). In all patients the fractures healed within the normal period, the colour of the skin was normal and hardly noticeable atrophy was found in 5 patients only. The above results are illustrated by the following example:

> A 24-year-old violinist had an accident involving his arm on March 16th, 1967. The arm was immobilised in plaster because of fracture of the neck of the humerus. The patient was admitted for prophylactic interferential therapy on April 18th, 1967. Fifteen treatments at a constant frequency of 100 Hz each were given daily over a period of 15 to 20 minutes. Control X-rays taken on May 6th, 1967 showed fracture consolidation. No muscle atrophy or joint rigidity was found after removal of immobilisation. The skin was normal in colour. The patient complained of mild pains only and 'a kind of weakness in the arm'. After 3 days of IT at a rhythmical frequency of 90–100 Hz and 0–100 Hz, the patient was discharged healthy and was able to continue his work as a violinist.

The above observations show that IT when applied during immobilisation, is a valuable preventive treatment against complications after fractures and shortens the time necessary for restoration of function.

Our systematic observations of 300 patients with different bone fractures also showed that IT helped to accelerate the elimination of sequelae such as painful rigidity of the joints, muscle atrophy and circulatory disorders (Nikolova, 1971a). Interferential therapy in these cases is applied at a rhythmical frequency of 0–100 Hz as it relieves pain and promptly regulates trophic disorders. A rhythmical frequency of 0–10/15 Hz is applied in stiff joints and for stimulation of muscles. In all cases IT is appropriately combined with massage, remedial exercises and baths at a temperature of 36°C.

Interferential therapy, especially in weak and

inactive patients, is the proper way to start active rehabilitation, since it does not require any physical effort. The period of recovery after long weeks of immobilisation can be significantly shortened.

Delayed callus formation

Consolidation, particularly in open fractures, can be delayed for different reasons. The most common are:

1. Insufficient blood supply in the vicinity of the fragments
2. A belated, incorrect or insufficient period of immobilisation
3. Infection in the fracture area
4. Interposition of soft tissues between fragments
5. General debility of the patient, e.g. avitaminosis

Lack of prophylactic measures during immobilisation also has unfavourable effects. For instance, none of the patients with delayed callus formation had the necessary prophylactic physiotherapy with IC or other appropriate physical treatments, such as ultraviolet rays, massage and exercises.

The effect of interferential therapy on bone tissue regeneration has been studied by us for 20 years. The following important conclusions have been drawn as a result of investigations carried out for the period from 1963 to 1970 on 300 patients aged between 8 and 76 years:

1. Interferential current of a constant frequency of 100 Hz stimulates formation of both endosteal and periosteal callus and can be applied in metal osteosynthesis (Nikolova, 1969b,d, 1970a,e).
2. Compared to physical methods used previously, such as US, syncardial pulses and electrophoresis with $CaCl_2$, IT yields far better results (Table 10.1). Its therapeutic effect is enhanced when combined with the appropriate drug treatment and remedial exercises.

The problem of stimulation of osteogenesis has always been one of the most significant in traumatology. It is a well-known fact that timely consolidation depends on a number of local and general factors. Of special importance, as has been stressed by many authors, is blood supply (Willengger, 1971; Hirthe, 1972). They all agree that if the circulation of blood and intercellular fluid in the fractured area is not normalised, the metabolism (hypoxia)[6] of bone fragments becomes unfavourable, interfering with the regener-

[6] Makley (1967) proved experimentally that chronic hypoxia leads to retarded bone regeneration.

Table 10.1 Effect of different physical methods on delayed callus formation

Applied therapeutic method	Number of patients	Therapeutic results*			
		Healthy	Greatly improved	Improved	No effect
IC	150	110(73%)	35(23%)	5(4%)	–
IT combined with drugs	60	48(80%)	12(20%)	–	–
Ultrasound	20	8(40%)	8(40%)	4(20%)	–
Syncardial pulses	20	8(40%)	9(45%)	3(15%)	–
Electrophoresis with $CaCl_2$	20	–	2(10%)	10(50%)	8(40%)
Ultraviolet radiation†	30	–	6(20%)	15(50%)	9(30%)

* 'Healthy' = complete consolidation shown on X-ray. Function was restored. 'Greatly improved' = considerable improvement shown on X-ray, but the line of fracture was still visible. The limb can function but caution and care are required. 'Improved' = consolidation was beginning (dim picture of the callus). The limb can function with the protection of a splint and an orthopaedic apparatus

† These data and the experience of other authors have shown that ultraviolet radiation and electrophoresis may be more important as a preventive measure against delayed callus formation

ation process. Mechanical rest,[7] which enables earlier vascularisation, is pointed out to be an essential advantage of metal osteosynthesis. With faulty internal fixation, vascular spasm occurs and results in a decrease in blood flow to the fracture area.

In 1962 Trueta proved that in spite of proper fixation, consolidation is retarded if the blood circulation is not restored. In general, all authors are of the opinion that the main reason for delayed callus formation and pseudoarthrosis is a haemodynamic disturbance in the area of the fracture. Tissue incompatibility is characterised on X-ray by accelerated resorption of the transplant or by retarded readjustment, and measures taken to ensure the proper vascularisation are, therefore, of essential importance.

Orthopaedic surgeons usually rely on metal fixation and immobilisation only, and do not resort to physical agents as a prophylactic measure in cases of delayed bone regeneration. Not all physical agents, however, are suitable for that purpose. It is well-known that local application of ultratherm (ultrahigh frequency), microwaves, decimetre waves and galvanic current is contraindicated in metal osteosynthesis (Arnold, 1978).

[7] Mechanical rest and close contact by internal fixation create optimal conditions for regeneration and allow early vascularisation. As has been pointed out by many authors, however, the process of osteogenesis can also be disturbed by internal fixation. In this case, IT at a constant frequency of 100 or 120 Hz (depending on the apparatus) is a valuable, harmless and accessible method.

Bearing in mind the above factors, we set ourselves the following tasks:

1. To extend the studies on IT in metal osteosynthesis and examine its effect in recent osteotomies.[8]
2. To study the influence of an application of IC alternating with US for possible improvement through mutual therapeutic effects in delayed callus formation.

A total of 307 patients have been under systematic observation, 250 with retarded callus formation (100 with metal osteosynthesis), 15 threatened by pseudoarthrosis, 30 operated on for pseudoarthrosis as sequelae to different fractures of long bones and 12 with recent osteotomies (Table 10.2). None of the patients had had any prophylactic physiotherapy during immobilisation. Drug treatment and physiotherapy carried out because of the delayed consolidation, including massage, ultraviolet radiation and electrophoresis with $CaCl_2$, had proved inefficient.

As in our former studies, IT in all patients was applied at a constant frequency of 100 Hz. The four electrodes were positioned so that the extremity involved was in the interference area of the two currents of medium frequency. Treatments were given daily over a period of 15 to 20 minutes.[9]

[8] Patients were diagnosed and sent for IT by the Institute of Orthopaedics and Traumatology in Sofia.
[9] The therapy in 60 patients was combined with drugs (Emdabol [tiomesterone], methandienone).

Table 10.2 Effect of IT on delayed callus formation with internal fixation and on recent osteotomies

Diagnosis	Number of patients	Therapeutic results*	
		Discharged healthy	Discharged with improvement
Delayed callus formation without metal osteosynthesis	150	110(73%)	40(27%)
Delayed callus formation in nailing osteosynthesis	100	79(79%)	21(21%)
Threatened by pseudoarthrosis	15	15(100%)	–
Pseudoarthrosis after osteotomy	30	13(43%)	17(57%)
Recent osteotomy	12	12(100%)	–

* 'Discharged with improvement' = with different degrees of improvement, established by X-ray

The therapeutic effect was assessed on the basis of the following indices: clinical findings (relieved or subsiding pain, absence or decrease of trophic disturbances), X-ray, oscillography and capillaroscopy in patients with upper extremity fracture. The results achieved are given in Table 10.2.

The 'healthy' group included patients with healing established clinically and by X-ray. X-ray analysis before and after treatment showed that IT in patients with metal osteosynthesis stimulates and leads to osteogenesis in 79% (Table 10.2), after an average of 20 to 40 treatments. Oscillographic investigations showed the highest values of the oscillographic index both after a single treatment and after completion of IT. Capillaroscopy showed that when stimulated by interferential current, the number of functioning capillaries per visual field increased ($p < 0.05$), which is in line with our observations on improvement of blood supply and metabolism (Nikolova & Davidov, 1979).

These data give us grounds to accept a relationship between improved blood supply due to interferential therapy (Fig. 10.5) and the obvious stimulation of callus formation. The analgesic effect of IC is also significant, and its

regulating influence on the metabolism of electrolytes, sodium, potassium and calcium plays an important role in protein biosynthesis. On the basis of our observations, wider application of IT can be recommended as an appropriate method for stimulation of callus formation in internal fixation (plates, clamps, Kuntscher nails). The following two examples illustrate this beneficial therapeutic effect:

A 38-year-old patient was in a car accident on August 15th, 1976. He sustained an olecranon fracture and soft tissue injuries. His arm was placed in a plaster slab. On September 2nd, 1976 he was operated on to allow nailing of the olecranon fragments. The X-ray taken on September 3rd, 1976 showed that the two fragments were well reduced and fixed. From September 18th hydrotherapy was conducted with underwater exercises, massage of the whole hand and remedial exercises, including forced passive movements (therapeutic fault!) for a total of 40 treatments. Then diadynamic current was applied.

The X-ray taken on November 13th, 1976 showed no evidence of callus formation. Nevertheless, treatment with massage and passive movements was continued, which ended in displacement of the fragments, without any callus formation. After the review examination, a second operation was considered, but following discussion of the case, the surgeons-traumatologists decided to carry out treatment with IC first.

The patient was admitted to our Clinic on January 27th, 1977 (165 days after the accident and 147 days after the operation) with a diagnosis of left-sided pseudo-

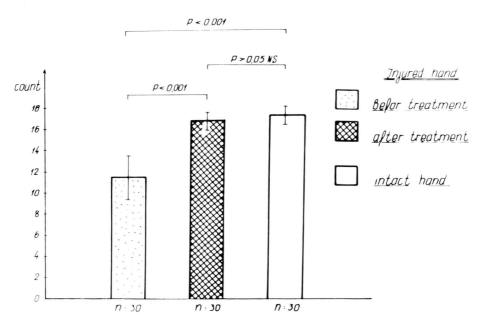

Fig. 10.5 Number of capillaries before and after treatment in patients with delayed callus formation.

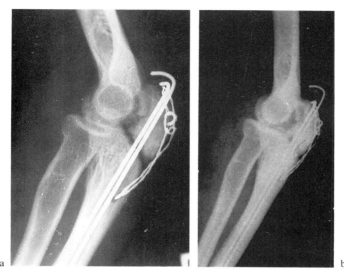

Fig. 10.6 Pseudoarthrosis of the olecranon. a. Before treatment.
b. After IT, showing consolidation of bone fragments.

arthrosis of the olecranon following fracture and internal
fixation (Fig. 10.6a). Sixty treatments with IC were
applied, which resulted in consolidation of bone (Fig.
10.6b) and restoration of function.

A 23-year-old patient was admitted to our Clinic with a
diagnosis of a fractured humerus with internal fixation
the 60th day after the operation and elbow contracture
(Fig. 10.8a–c). Twenty-five treatments with IC were
applied resulting in good consolidation (Fig. 10.7c,d) and
function restoration (Fig. 10.8d–f).

Recent osteotomy

Interferential therapy has been used since
1974/1975 prophylactically as early as the second
day after operation. Twelve patients were under
our observation (1 man and 11 women), 4 of them
aged between 20 and 30, 6 between 31 and 50 and
2 between 51 and 70. Eleven patients had
dysplastic arthrosis of the hip and 1 a *traumatic* one
(after fracture of the femoral neck). Varus
osteotomy with derotation was performed in 10
patients, valgus osteotomy in 1 and McMurray's
osteotomy in 1 patient.

Treatment with IC was applied at a constant
frequency of 100 Hz for 20 minutes daily, for a
total 12, 15 or 20 treatments. The postoperative
period in all patients was uneventful and the
wound healed normally. Callus was formed
within 25 to 30 days on average, which made it
possible to place a load on the extremity as

soon as the end of the first month. Nine
patients were discharged without contracture,
and 3 with flexion contracture up to between 10°
and 15°.

It is noteworthy that our observations in 1979
were confirmed by Güttler & Kleiditzsch (1979)
who found more rapid callus formation in rabbits
subjected to IC compared to the controls. Later,
Kleiditzsch (1982), when comparing the influence
of a current of rectangular pulses with that of IC at
a constant frequency of 100 Hz in experimental
osteotomy, pointed out that IC promoted bone
mineralisation. Laabs et al (1980), on the basis of
experimental studies, also reported that IT stimulates healing of fractures since it accelerates
mineralisation without leading to ectopic mineralisation or other side effects. It is therefore
advisable to apply IC for a prophylactic purpose in
patients with recent osteotomy to accelerate the
healing process.

Consecutive application of IC and US in delayed callus formation

The effect of the consecutive application of IC
and ultrasound in delayed callus formation was
studied from 1977 to 1980. Our observations
cover a total of 40 patients (26 men and 14
women) with the following age distribution: 1

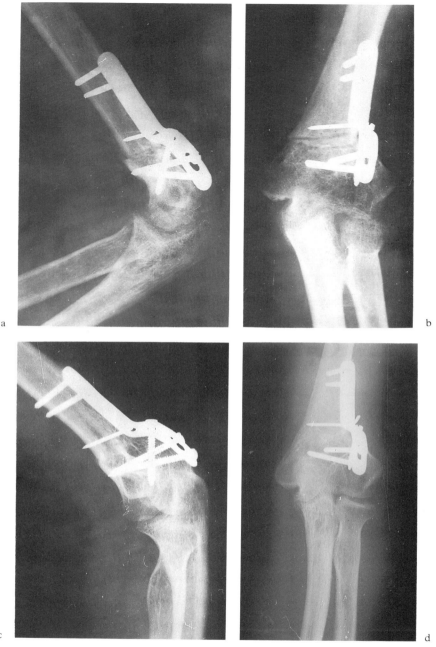

Fig. 10.7 Patient's condition on X-ray after metal osteosynthesis. a,b. Before treatment with IC. c,d. After treatment, showing complete consolidation.

patient aged 16, 12 patients between 21 and 40, 25 patients between 41 and 60 and 2 patients over 70. The time which elapsed from the day of the fracture to admission to our Clinic is given in

Table 10.3: 65% of the patients were sent after the 3rd or the 6th month.

Fourteen patients sustained fractures of the bones of the upper extremity, and 26 fractures of

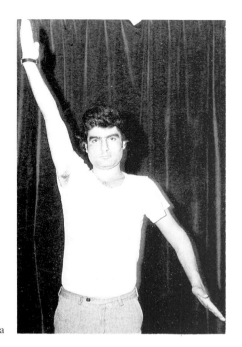

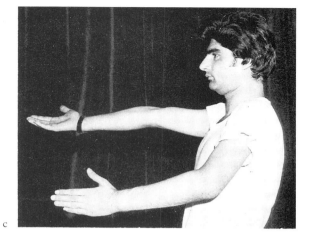

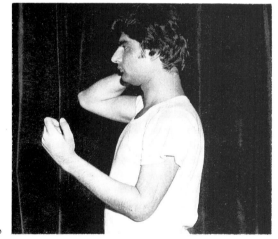

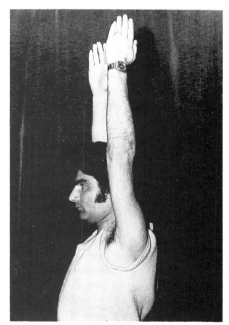

Fig. 10.8 Patient's functional ability. a,b,c. Before IT.
d,e,f. Functional repair after IT.

Fig. 10.8 f. overleaf.

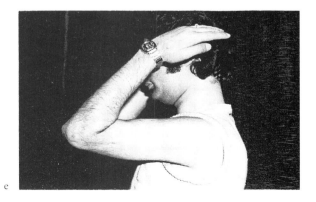

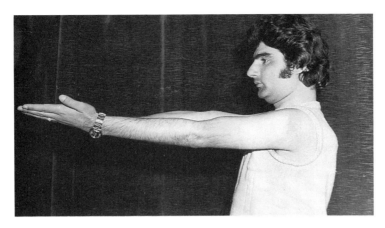

Fig. 10.8 f

Table 10.3 Time lapse between fracture and consecutive treatment with IT and US in delayed callus formation

Interval between fracture and start of treatment	Number of patients
45–60 days	4(10%)
60–90 days	10(25%)
91–180 days	23(57.5%)
181–380 days	3(7.5%)

the lower extremity. Poor reduction was found in 4 patients, 3 had nail fixation and 2 Sudeck's atrophy. Interferential current was applied in each case of delayed callus formation at a constant frequency of 100 Hz, and immediately after each treatment US was performed using the labile technique at a dosage of 0.2–0.4 W/cm^2, for 6 to 12 minutes, depending on the affected area.[10] The results obtained after an average of 20 to 25 treatments are given in Table 10.4. They indicate

[10] It has been found experimentally that when applied at that dosage on the 2nd or 3rd day after fracture, US stimulates osteogenesis.

a somewhat higher percentage of patients discharged as 'healthy', i.e. with recovery established clinically and on X-ray, than in the case of patients subjected to IC only (cf Table 10.1). The beneficial effect of combined treatment is also much more pronounced than in the isolated application of US (Fig. 10.9) which led to complete recovery in only 40% of our patients (cf Table 10.1) (Nikolova, 1969, 1971).

Function was also restored in patients with nail fixation, which confirms the opinion of some authors that US in small dosage has no harmful effect on tissues in such cases.

The results of the consecutive application of IC and US are illustrated by the following examples:

A 54-year-old patient had an accident on May 10th, 1977 and sustained fractures of the two bones of the left forearm. After reduction the forearm and hand were immobilised in a plaster cast. The control X-ray on the 20th day following the injury showed poor alignment, which necessitated repeated reduction. Plaster immobilisation lasted for a total of 5 months with continuous pain in the area of the fracture.

Table 10.4 Results of the consecutive application of IT and US in delayed callus formation

Number of patients	Therapeutic results*	
	Discharged healthy	Discharged improved
40	35(87.5%)	5(12.5%)

* 'Discharged healthy' = recovery established clinically and on X-ray.
  'Discharged improved' = considerable improvement on X-ray, although line of fracture is visible

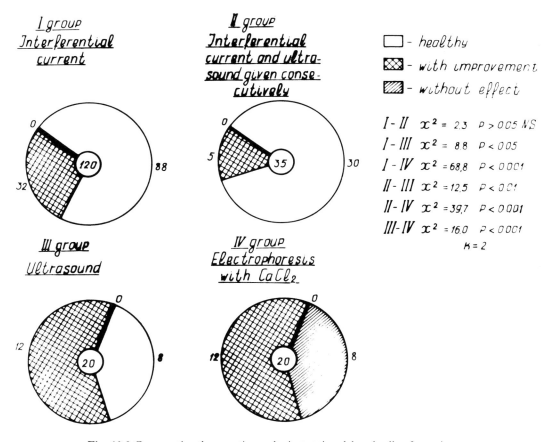

Fig. 10.9 Comparative therapeutic results in treating delayed callus formation.

On October 27th, 1977 the patient was admitted for surgical treatment, but as callus formation had already started, the plaster was removed and the patient was sent to our Clinic on November 21st, 1977. The diagnosis was delayed callus formation following left-sided fractures of the radius and ulna — Sudeck's atrophy (2nd stage) — and elbow joint contracture (Figs 10.10 and 10.11). Interferential therapy combined with US was applied, which led to complete healing of the fractures and restoration of function (Figs 10.10 and 10.11).

A student had an accident on June 16th, 1979 and sustained a fracture of the left humerus in the proximal metaphysis. The arm was placed in plaster. After removal of the plaster he was sent to our Clinic on August 20th of the same year with the following complaints: delayed callus formation (the fracture line did not show spread of trabecular bone from the surrounding area), signs of frozen shoulder and painful rigidity in the adjacent elbow joint (Figs 10.12 and 10.13). Interferential therapy conducted in turn with US resulted in complete repair of function within 20 days (Fig. 10.13). X-rays taken on November 13th, 1979 indicated union of the fracture.

A 39-year-old patient sustained a fractured arm on August 2nd, 1976. After reduction, the fragments were

immobilised. The plaster was removed on January 11th, 1977. He was admitted to our Clinic on the 21st January of the same year (5 months after the fracture) with a diagnosis of fracture-dislocation of the radius and ulna, non-union with a tendency to pseudarthrosis formation and Sudeck's atrophy 2nd-3rd stage (Fig. 10.14). Moderately pronounced osteoporosis was also found in the bones of the left elbow joint. Interferential therapy was carried out in turn with US, the results of which are indicated in Figure 10.15. All movements possible were restored as far as they could go. Nothing more could be achieved without operative intervention.

Small bone fragments (comminuted fracture)

These are comparatively common in various types of bone injuries. The chance of union in this type of fracture remains problematical. Comminuted fractures often result in pseudarthrosis. Our studies (Nikolova & Ignatov, 1969; Nikolova, 1971a, 1979) showed excellent results using IC at

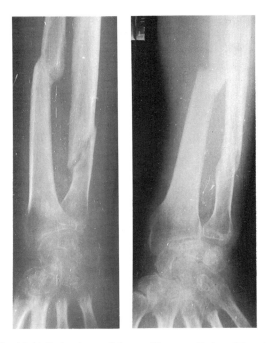

a   b

Fig. 10.10 Patient's condition on X-ray. a. Before IT and US treatment (6 months after the fracture). b. After treatment, showing repair of the bone structure.

a constant frequency of 100 Hz both in restoring function and in achieving union. This beneficial effect is observed even in malalignment of the basic fracture, as well as in concomitant complications, such as Sudeck's atrophy and delayed union. The results are better when IT is started immediately after removal of fixation.

The following laboratory and biochemical indices were established in 150 patients before and after treatment:[11] leukocyte count, sedimentation rate (after Westergreen), serum calcium and phosphorus level and their relationship and amounts of K, Na, Cl, plasma protein, sialic acid, alkaline phosphatase and fibrinogen, all of them being within normal limits with statistically insignificant differences after treatment. The lack of change in the parameters examined[12] makes us think that IC contributes to the elimination of haemodynamic disorders in the area of the

fracture and tissue hypoxia. Interferential current effectively stimulates osteogenesis, leading to normalisation of metabolic processes in the traumatised bone tissue.

The results obtained from these observations over a 20-year period have led to the following important conclusions:

1. Interferential current stimulates the formation of both endosteal and periosteal callus. In this respect it is superior to other physiotherapeutic methods applied so far. The stimulating effect of IC on osteogenesis is enhanced when combined with relevant drugs or ultrasound therapy.
2. Interferential current, when applied with a prophylactic purpose as early as the first days after fracture, usually leads to timely consolidation of the fracture and prevents complications such as contractures and loss of function. An essential advantage is that it can be applied in the presence of metal implants.

Sudeck's atrophy (acute traumatic osteoporosis)

This condition, described by Sudeck in 1900, has been given various names the most common being Sudeck's atrophy (osteoporosis). However, a number of authors (Glick & Helal, 1976) consider the name *algo-neurodystrophy* to be most suitable, as this includes three aspects of the disease: pain, a neurogenic mechanism of onset and dystrophic symptoms. As compared with spotty bone dystrophy, the aetiology of the disease has not yet been completely clarified. The various theories can be included under the following headings: inflammatory, inactivating, mechanical, neurogenic, neurohumoral and vascular. Changes in blood circulation and permeability are considered by most authors to be the main sign of the disease. All tissues are involved both locally and in the vicinity of the lesion, except the joint cartilage and tendons (Gremieux, 1975).

Several methods have been proposed for treatment of Sudeck's atrophy but none is generally accepted so far. Most authors point out that clinical recovery is slow — 5 to 6 months on

[11] Most of the patients (i.e. 110 or 73%) were admitted 3 months after the fracture.
[12] And the pronounced vasodilating effect of IC proven by capillaroscopic, rheographic and histochemical examinations.

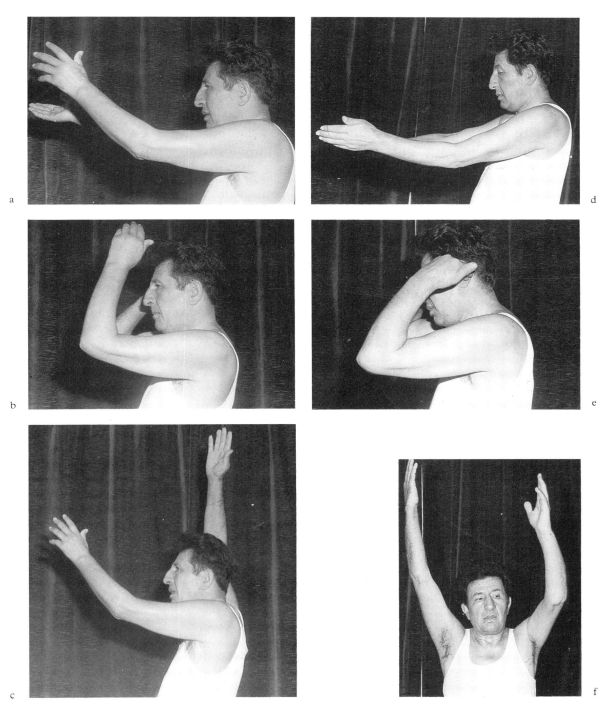

Fig. 10.11 Patient's functional ability. a,b,c. Before IC and US treatment. d,e,f. Functional repair after treatment.

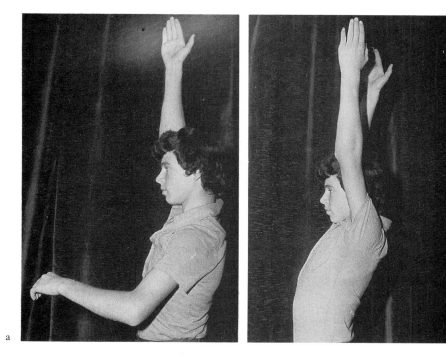

a   b

Fig. 10.12 Patient with frozen shoulder in retarded callus formation. a. Before treatment. b. After treatment.

average — and that the X-ray picture becomes normal much later. Complete recovery is considered impossible by some authors, if the process has reached the 3rd stage (Gremieux, 1975; Portias, 1977). This is accounted for by the complex aetiopathogenesis of the disease and often by the malunion of the fractures, long-term immobilisation and inappropriate thermotherapy.

Interferential current was introduced by us at a constant frequency of 100 Hz (Nikolova, 1964) on the following grounds:

1. IC at the above frequency has a strong analgesic effect and is effective in the treatment of acute traumatic osteoporosis.

2. IC regulates the vascular tone, and more particularly it helps to normalise the microcirculation. A number of authors have found a fall in the count of visible capillaries and blood flow rate in the 2nd stage of dystrophy (Schlosser, 1973).

3. IC improves metabolism, ensures better oxygen supply to tissues, increases the lymph flow and shifts the pH to the alkaline side, which is of essential importance as tissue acidosis in the dystrophic area has been established by many authors.

Interferential therapy is applied in the following manner: 4-plate electrodes of an area of 50 or 100 cm^2 are positioned so that the dystrophy area is in the interference zone of the two medium-frequency currents. The first two electrodes are situated paravertebrally in the segmental area, and the other two in the distal part of the affected limb. Treatments are given daily for 15 to 20 minutes, the current power depending on the patient's sensitivity: a sensation of slight vibrating massage should be experienced (6–25 mA is used, on average). Fifteen to 25 or more treatments are required with a few days' break to prevent the tissue adapting to the stimulation.

From 1963 to the end of 1977 IC was applied in

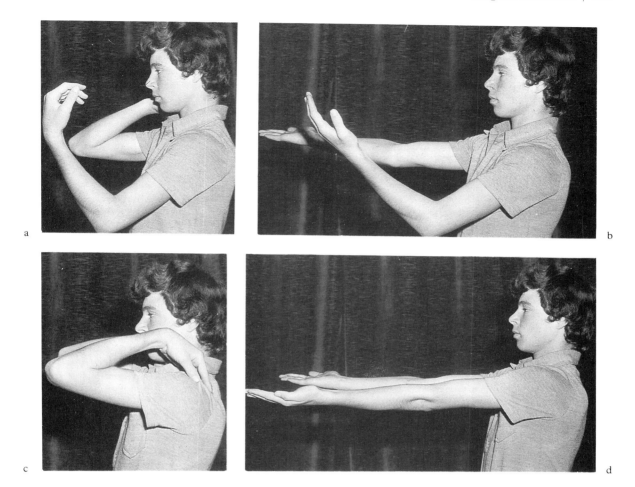

Fig. 10.13 Patient's functional ability. a,b. Before treatment with IC and US. c,d. After treatment, showing functional repair.

400 patients with acute traumatic osteoporosis. Their sex and age distribution are shown in Table 10.5, confirming the opinion of many authors that the highest incidence of the disease occurs above the age of 40, mainly in women. The primary aetiological factors which led to dystrophy are given in Table 10.6, from which it is seen that Sudeck's atrophy usually develops after fracture of the radius in the typical area (Colles' fracture): in those attending our Clinic it accounted for 158 patients or 45%. Some other aetiological factors are:

1. Malalignment — 88 patients (25%) — most often in those with Colles' fracture of the radius.
2. Energetic thermotherapy (paraffin application, ultratherm, microwaves, hot baths) immediately after removal of the immobilisation, i.e. before the dystrophy had developed — 308 patients (77%).

Table 10.5 Sex and age distribution of patients with Sudeck's atrophy

Men	Women	21–40 years	41–60 years	61–75 years
182	218	102	238	60

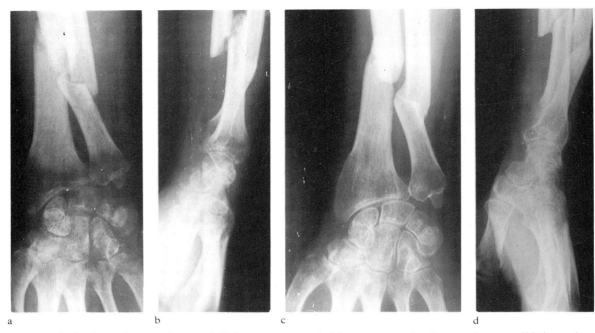

Fig. 10.14 Patient's condition on X-ray. a,b. Before treatment. c,d. After treatment, showing complete consolidation and removal of the signs of Sudeck's atrophy.

Table 10.6 Aetiological factors in patients with Sudeck's atrophy

Primary aetiology	Number of patients	Location of fracture	Number of patients
Bone fractures	350	shoulder bone (humerus)	9(3%)
		ulna and radius	4(1%)
		radius (lower end) (Colles')	158(45%)
		navicular bone	12(3.5%)
		neck of femur	3(1%)
		tibia and fibula	48(14%)
		medial and lateral malleoli fractures	60(17%)
		variety of foot bones	56(16%)
Injuries of the joints, contusion, sprains, dislocation	50		

The patients were also distributed according to the stage of the disease, and these figures are given in Table 10.7. Sudeck's atrophy was

Table 10.7 Stage of Sudeck's atrophy

Stage of disease	Number of patients
1st	52
2nd	275
3rd	73

accompanied by delayed callus formation in 65 patients, 16 of them with internal fixation.

Previous treatment with Novocain block, various drugs, diadynamic current and iontophoresis with $CaCl_2$ in 86 patients was ineffective.

Out-patient IT was given to all our patients.[13]

[13] Schlosser (1973), Gremieux (1975), Portias (1977) and others prefer hospital in-patient treatment, which enables an elevated position of the extremity and precise estimation of the therapeutic procedures necessary. In-patient treatment with IC is generally not required.

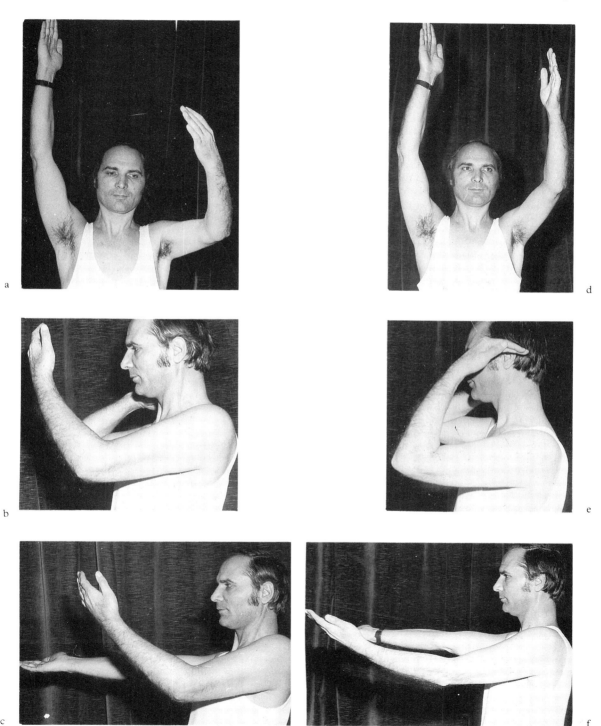

Fig. 10.15 Patient's functional ability. a,b,c. Before IT and US treatment. d,e,f. After treatment, showing maximum repair of function.

In 80 of the patients it was combined with suitable drugs (nicotinyl alcohol, bamethan sulphate, kallidinogenase) to help healing, especially in patients with malalignment (Nikolova, 1971a, 1979). Remedial exercises were applied in all patients after the pain subsided. Clinical symptoms of the disease (pain, trophic disturbances, rigidity of joints) disappeared within 16 to 60 days, depending on the stage at which treatment was started.

Best results were achieved in the 1st stage of the disease, and worst in the 3rd stage. Comparative studies with other physiotherapeutic methods (using clinical and X-ray examination) showed that the best results were achieved from the application of IC. Special attention was paid to changes in the X-ray picture and to the capillary findings after IT had been applied.

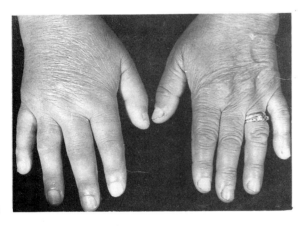

a

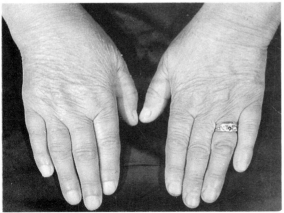

b

Fig. 10.16 Patient with Sudeck's atrophy of the right hand. a. Before IC treatment. b. After IC treatment.

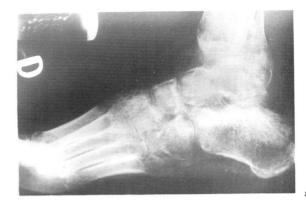

a

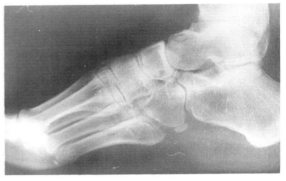

b

Fig. 10.17 Patient with Sudeck's atrophy of the foot. a. X-ray before treatment. b. X-ray after IT, showing normalisation.

The following examples illustrate the excellent results obtained with IT:

A 69-year-old patient was admitted with a diagnosis of post Colles' fracture, 2nd stage Sudeck's atrophy. A total of 20 treatments was applied. The results are presented in Figure 10.16a,b.

Another patient was admitted with a diagnosis of post fracture Sudeck's atrophy. The IC treatments led to normalisation of the X-ray image, as seen in Figure 10.17b.

A 55-year-old patient fell down on her right arm on March 18th, 1972. She was given X-ray reduction of fracture and plaster immobilisation of the hand. During immobilisation she had severe pain and oedema of the fingers, which necessitated removal of the plaster. Then the arm was once more put in plaster and remained so until June 8th, 1972.

She was admitted to our Clinic on June 17th, 1972, i.e. 3 months after the fracture, with a diagnosis of right post Colles' fracture and cervical arthrosis. In addition to being hypersensitive, she had Sudeck's atrophy at the 2nd-3rd stage (Fig. 10.18a) and frozen shoulder. Pronounced trophic changes were apparent, movements were restricted (Fig. 10.19a–d) and the pain was so unbearable that the patient spoke of suicide. Interferential therapy was applied and after the pain subsided it was applied in combination with remedial exercises. The X-ray became normal (Fig. 10.18b), and the function of the hand was restored (Fig. 10.19e–h).

A 38-year-old medical worker had a car accident on September 25th, 1980 in which she sustained a severe injury of the right leg. The X-ray showed trimalleolar fractures (3rd degree Pott's) of the right leg. Manual reduction proved ineffective, so the leg was placed in traction for 50 days. The control X-ray did not show any change in the condition. A repeated manual reduction was performed under anaesthesia, followed by plaster immobilisation for a further 90 days. After removal of the plaster a marked hypotrophy of the leg was observed with oedema of the foot which increased in the standing position, numbness in the toes, contracture of the first toe and markedly restricted and painful movements in the ankle joint. Treatment was carried out with ultrasound, salt baths and remedial exercises but her condition deteriorated. She walked with crutches without stepping

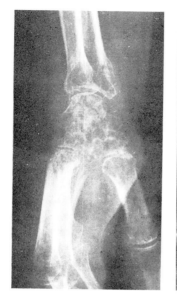
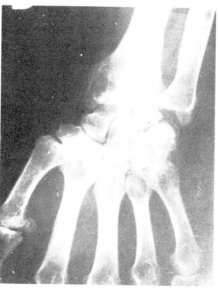

a   b

Fig. 10.18 Patient with Sudeck's atrophy — 2nd-3rd stage. a. X-ray before treatment with IC. b. X-ray after treatment, showing normalisation of the X-ray image.

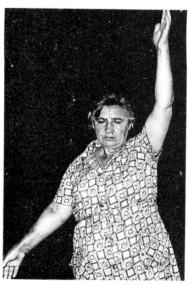
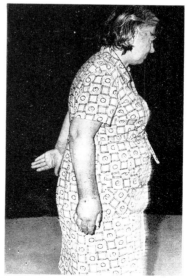

a   b

Fig. 10.19 Same patient as in Figure 10.18. a,b,c,d. Before treatment. (Contd. overleaf)

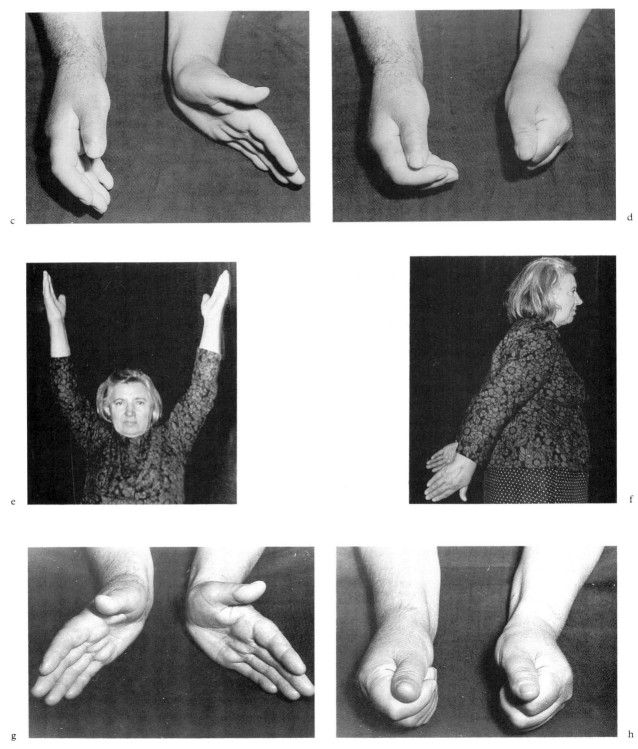

Fig. 10.19 (contd.) Same patient as in Figure 10.18. e,f,g,h. After IC treatment, showing functional repair.

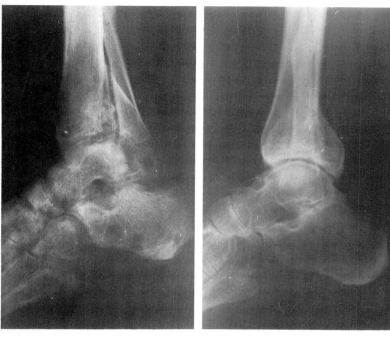

a   b

Fig. 10.20 Patient with Sudeck's atrophy of the foot — 7 months after the fracture. a. X-ray before treatment. b. X-ray after IC treatment, showing normalisation of bone structure.

onto the affected limb. The control X-ray on March 14th, 1981, i.e. about 7 months after the fracture, gave a diagnosis of right 3rd degree Pott's fracture with 2nd and 3rd stage Sudeck's atrophy and a fractured navicula (Fig. 10.20a).

Interferential therapy was applied in combination with remedial exercises. The control X-ray did not show even a late phenomenon of Sudeck's atrophy. No hypertrophic osteoporosis was observed. The structure was homogenous, the small trabeculae were of fine structure and normal density (Fig. 10.20b). The fracture of the navicula was consolidated. Narrowing of the talo-navicular joint space is visible as a residual phenomenon due to imperfect orthopaedic treatment. Function was restored and the patient returned to her work as a nurse.

A 52-year-old mine technician had an accident on April 3rd, 1981. The X-ray revealed fractures of the two bones of the forearm with severe dislocation of the fragments and subluxation of the 1st metacarpo-phalangeal joint of the right thumb. Open reduction with intramedullary nailing of the radius was carried out and a plaster slab applied for 12 days (until removal of the stiches), followed by immobilisation in an all round plaster for 5 months. The X-ray check-up on August 31st, 1981 showed incomplete consolidation of the bones of the right forearm, slight dislocation, avulsion of the ulnar styloid process, and marked osteoporosis in the distal parts of the radius and the elbow, especially pronounced in the area of the carpal and metacarpal bones (Fig. 10.21). The plaster was removed and surgical treatment was recommended.

The patient refused the operation. He was admitted to

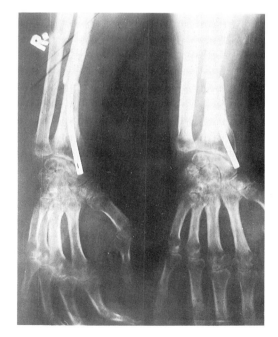

Fig. 10.21 X-ray of patient after intramedullary nailing, showing retarded callus formation, Sudeck's atrophy (2nd stage) — before IT.

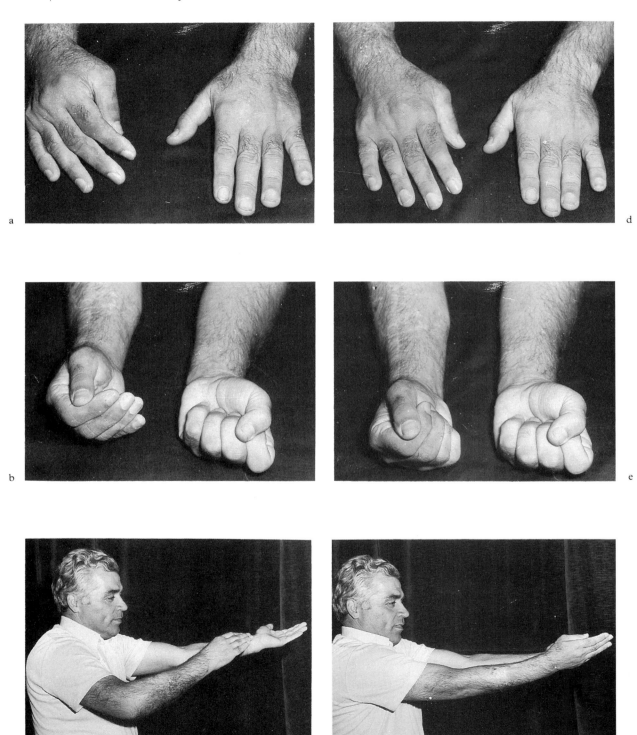

Fig. 10.22 Same patient as in Figure 10.22. a,b,c. Before IT treatment. d,e,f. After treatment, showing functional repair.

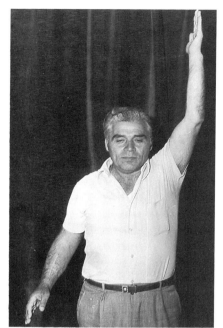

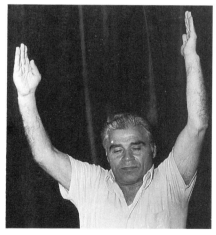

Fig. 10.22 (contd.) g. Before IT treatment, h. After treatment, showing functional repair.

our Clinic with a diagnosis of multiple fractures of the right radius and ulna with intramedullary nailing, delayed consolidation and 2nd stage Sudeck's atrophy. The movements of the arm (shoulder, elbow and wrist) were affected and rather painful, and marked trophic changes in the forearm were observed (Fig. 10.22a–d).

Out-patient IT with remedial exercises resulted in good consolidation of the broken bones, relief of Sudeck's atrophy and restoration of function of the arm and wrist. The patient was discharged after 2 months in very good condition (Fig. 10.22e–h).

Influence of IC on X-ray appearance

The assertion of some authors that X-ray appearance becomes normal very slowly without occurring in all cases and our findings of improved X-ray pictures after only 15 to 20 days of IT in some patients, gave us grounds to study the reverse evolution of Sudeck's atrophy. For this purpose 150 patients were followed up (Nikolova & Balchev, 1977). An X-ray of all patients was taken before treatment — 20 in the 1st stage, 95 in the 1st-2nd and 2nd stage and 35 in the 2nd-3rd and 3rd stage. Check-up X-rays were taken on the 20th day, 1, 2, 4 and 6 months and 1 to 3 years after treatment, i.e. until the X-ray picture essentially improved or became normal. Analysis of the radiographs showed:

1. Restoration of a normal X-ray appearance is almost simultaneous with clinical recovery. The contours of the cortex, the disturbed structure of the cancellous substance and the abnormal consistency of the bone substance became normal within 30 days on average for patients in the 1st stage (Fig. 10.23). The time for repair was almost the same for patients in the 2nd stage (30 to 50 days). For patients in the 2nd-3rd stage and the 3rd stage, recovery occurred within 2 to 3 months on average (Figs 10.24 and 10.25). Lacunar, especially coarse-lacunar dystrophy was most persistent, with the X-ray picture becoming normal by the 3rd or 4th month. By the 5th month the fine bone structure was approximately the same as the intact extremity.

2. In patients who came long after the onset of Sudeck's syndrome as well as patients who had been given a wrong treatment for months, sharp and rough, subchondrally located dystrophic lacunae kept obtruding through the bony area, which could not regain its fine structure and normal consistency until the 6th month. Complete repair, however, was found in these patients as well within 1 to 2 years. The bone structure was repaired and the X-ray picture did not show any trace of the disease.

3. We noted in particular the fact that the X-ray picture became normal within the same

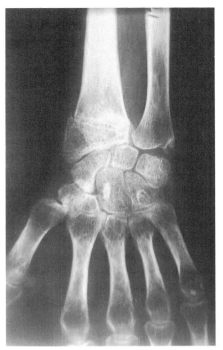 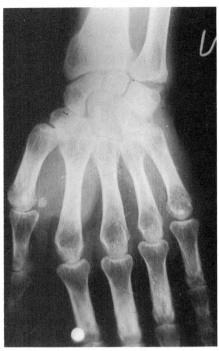

a   b

Fig. 10.23 Patient with 1st stage Sudeck's atrophy. a. X-ray before IT, showing diffuse osteoporotic process in the carpal areas, more pronounced in the metaphyseal areas of the metacarpus and the phalanges. Noteworthy is a sharp delineation of a bone island in the capitate, which contrasts with the osteoporotic background. b. X-ray after IT, showing normalisation of the bone structure in both the carpus and the metaphyseal area of the metacarpals. The island is hardly visible as its structure falls in line with the repaired density of the carpal bones. The fracture line, which is clearly outlined in Sudeck's atrophy, has disappeared and complete consolidation has taken place.

period, both in poor reductions of fractures and in dislocations, e.g. poor reduction of fragments in Dupuytren's and Colles' fractures in which the anatomical fault maintains and deepens the dystrophic changes, and in well-set fractures.

Observations of changes in the X-ray appearance in Sudeck's atrophy led to the following important practical conclusions:

1. Healing of bone lesions in patients with Sudeck's atrophy having undergone rehabilitation with IC is almost parallel with relief of clinical symptoms (pain, oedema, trophic disturbances, rigidity of the joints) and occurs in considerably shorter time than with methods applied so far — e.g. within 1 month (1st stage osteoporosis), within 2 to 4 months (2nd and 3rd stage

osteoporosis). Some authors (Mucha et al, 1984) in cases of Sudeck's atrophy of the hand, give priority to remedial exercises and do not apply IT. They experience much longer periods of recovery — 18 to 46 weeks — and do not indicate precisely the state of X-ray changes.

2. The repair process is markedly shortened in patients with poorly reduced fractures, which are considered to have the most unfavourable course in Sudeck's atrophies.

3. One advantage of the method is that patients are not obliged to stay in hospital when treated with IC.

IC and disorders of microcirculation

Capillaroscopy is widely applied in the diagnosis and treatment, and the temporary invalidity

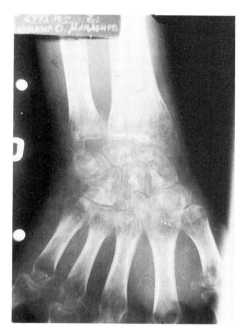
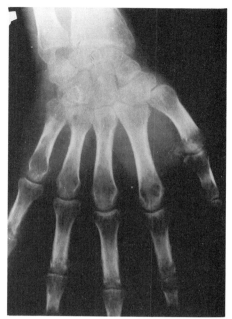

a
b

Fig. 10.24 Patient with 3rd stage Sudeck's atrophy. a. X-ray before IT, showing marked crushed structure of the small carpal bones, pronounced osteoporosis in the radius and ulna epiphyses and spotted structure of the spongy substance. The metaphyseal areas (well visible) of the five carpal bones and part of the phalanges are affected by pronounced osteoporosis, while the diaphyses of the same bones are not yet involved in the dystrophy. The small bones are more damaged, the contour being interrupted in certain spots with lacunar and cystic formations abounding inside. b. X-ray after IT, showing that the areas of epiphyseal osteoporotic alterations have significantly decreased and that the spongy structure of both the epiphyseal areas and the small bones of the carpus has become homogenous — manifest sign of recovery.

examination, for patients with Sudeck's atrophy as it gives valuable data on peripheral haemodynamics and microcirculation. A number of authors (Harff, 1957; Scheibe, 1960; Thorban, 1962) have studied the condition of microcirculation in acute traumatic osteoporosis (Sudeck's atrophy 1st to 3rd stage). The following changes were found:

1. In the acute stage there is a dilation and rise in the number of capillaries
2. In the dystrophic stage there is strong closure and a fall in the count of visible capillaries and in blood flow rate
3. In the stage of atrophy there is stricture, and a decrease in the count of visible capillaries and in blood flow rate

According to Thorban (1962) this capillary finding — the gross vascular changes — accounts for the fact that complete recovery is almost unattainable in long-term Sudeck's atrophy. The blood supply to the distal parts of the limbs is inadequate and cannot provide normal tissue nutrition.

The dynamics of the capillaroscopic condition of patients with Sudeck's atrophy had not yet been studied when we began our investigations. We have examined a total of 70 patients — 30 in the 1st stage and 40 in the 2nd stage. The state of the capillaries was taken on the nail bed of the 4th finger of both hands at a magnification of 80 (ocular No 8, object-glass No 10). The staining of the background, the count of functioning capillaries, their type and the halo and turbidity degree of the pericapillary space were all taken into consideration. The norm was accepted to be a pink background, 16–20 capillary loops per visual field, visible circulation of blood flow and the presence of halo and pericapillary space turbidity of the 1st degree. For clarity 4 types of capillary

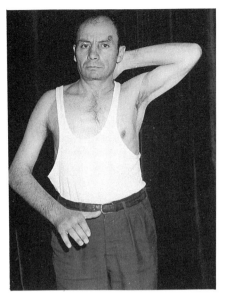

a

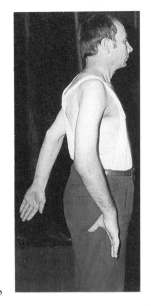

b

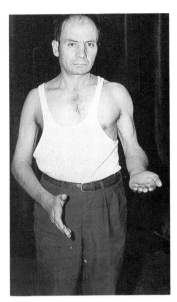

c

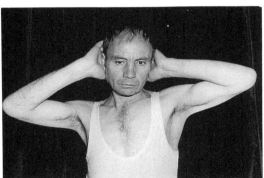

d

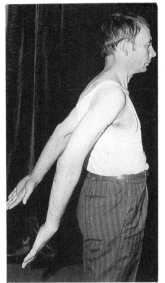

e

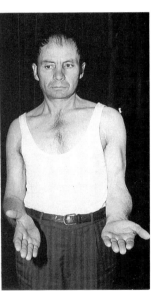

f

Fig. 10.25 Same patient as in Figure 10.24. a,b,c. Before IC treatment. d,e,f. After treatment, showing functional repair.

state were determined: normal, spastic, spastic-atonic and atonic.

A comparison of the results from the left and right hands made it possible to establish asymmetry (affected hand/intact hand) in the state of the capillaries of all patients under investigation.

We found dilation and increase in the numbers of capillaries in 1st stage patients. After

treatment, however, the asymmetry as compared with the intact hand was removed (Fig. 10.26).

The generalised capillaroscopic picture of the affected hand before treatment in 2nd stage patients was characterised by a predominant pale yellow (22.5%) and pale pink (55%) background, a reduced capillary count (per visual field) (Fig.

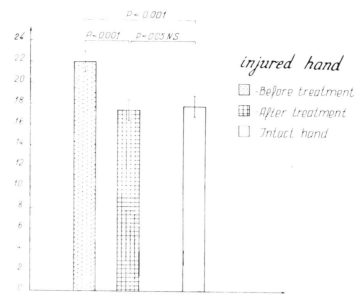

Fig. 10.26 Capillaries' count in 1st stage Sudeck's atrophy.

10.27), spastic or spastic-atonic capillaries, absent or fine-grained blood flow and marked pericapillary turbidity. This is suggestive of the presence of autonomic dystonia with sympathetic tone prevailing. Statistically significant normotonic dynamics in all parameters were established after treatment, as illustrated in Figures 10.28–10.33.

The normotonic dynamics in the capillaroscopic parameters under IT is a manifestation of an improved circulatory mechanism and vascular-tissue metabolism in the microcirculation of the patients under investigation.

The changes established give us grounds to consider capillaroscopy as an objective method which can be used in the diagnosis, examination of temporary invalidity and evaluation of a given therapy in patients with Sudeck's atrophy.

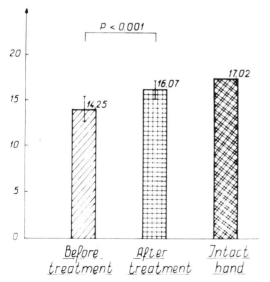

Fig. 10.27 Capillaries' count in 2nd stage Sudeck's atrophy.

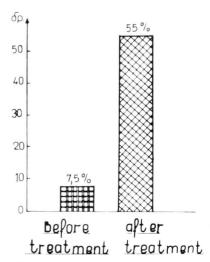

Fig. 10.28 Normal capillaries.

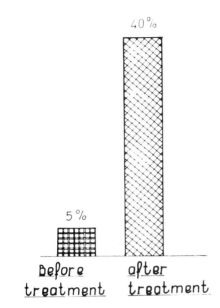

Fig. 10.29 Normal blood flow.

Rheographic examination of the affected and intact palm in 20 patients with 2nd stage Sudeck's atrophy before treatment showed vascular dystonia in the dystrophic area manifested by decreased elasticity and increased tone of capillaries, precapillary sphincters, arterioles and small arteries, with increased blood flow resistance and reduced blood supply. The rheographic changes were in accord with capillaroscopic data. Unidirectional normodynamics of rheographic indices such as elimination (removal) of capillary spasm and normalisation of pathologically disturbed haemodynamics in the dystrophic area were found as a result of the treatment (Figs 10.34 and 10.35).

Oscillographic investigation in over 100 patients before treatment showed pronounced asymmetry in the arterial tone and smoothing of asymmetry after IT.

Comparison of the clinical features and the X-ray findings with those of the oscillation index, capillaroscopy and rheography shows that elimination of asymmetry in these indices is directly related to the therapeutic effect, i.e. removal of asymmetry in the vascular tone is observed together with restoration of function and improvement of the X-ray appearance.

Comparative analysis of the effect of IT, ultrasound, syncardial massage and diadynamic current, showed that IT gave the most convincing results where other methods had failed (Nikolova, 1971a, 1983).[14,15]

The data obtained by us undoubtedly prove the beneficial effect of IT in Sudeck's atrophy and are suggestive of enhanced fixation of Ca ions in the affected dystrophic area. The proved effectiveness of IC in stimulating callus formation testifies to the same quality (Nikolova, 1969b,d,e,f, 1971a, 1979; Güttler & Kleiditzsch, 1979; Laabs, 1982a,b).

All authors point out the importance of early remedial exercises in patients with Sudeck's atrophy and recommend the inclusion of the affected extremity in the exercises as soon as the acute stage is over (Gremieux, 1975; Nikolova, 1979). Interferential therapy is therefore of great value not only because it removes microcirculatory disturbances, but also because it enables remedial exercises to be carried out at an earlier stage through the rapid relief of pain. This is of essential importance in preventing irreversible bone and other changes.

[14] In 50 patients before and after IT the following parameters were also followed up: erythrocyte sedimentation rate (after Westergreen), plasma protein, albumin, α_1, α_2, β and γ -globulin, sialic acid, Na, potassium, Ca, phosphorus (and their correlations), AP, chlorides. They were within normal limits in all patients, with statistically insignificant differences after treatment ($p > 0.05$). A rise of fibrinogen values was found in 17 patients (34%). $\times = 494.08$ before treatment and $\times = 421.33$ after treatment, the difference being statistically insignificant ($p > 0.05$).

[15] The condition of the neuromuscular apparatus was examined in 50 patients without concomitant lesion of the peripheral nerve by routine electrodiagnosis. Quantitative reduction of electroexcitability was found in 46 patients, and after treatment the asymmetry in the damaged hand became the same as in the intact one. EMG examination in 20 patients in the 1st, 2nd and 3rd stage of Sudeck's atrophy, showed no pathological denervation activity, the rate of conductivity and the distal latent time being within normal limits.

These results also give us ground to consider that local disorders of blood circulation, such as increased sympathetic tone and metabolic disturbances of various aetiology, play an important part in the onset of Sudeck's atrophy. Hence the necessity of applying methods enabling the normalisation of microcirculation and improvement of metabolic processes in the affected area. This is of the utmost importance, as healing of diffuse osteoporosis is impossible without eliminating tissue acidosis and ensuring normal tissue nutrition.

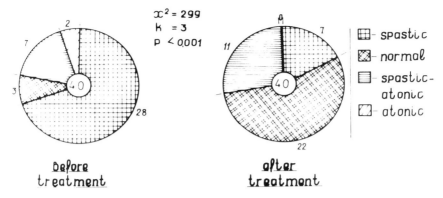

Fig. 10.30 Count and motility of the capillaries.

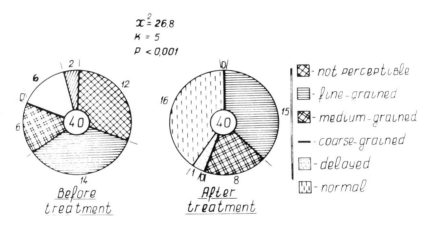

Fig. 10.31 Blood flow changes.

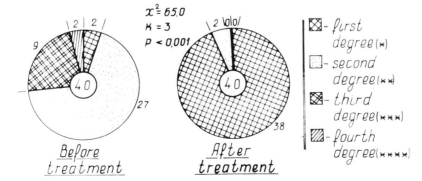

Fig. 10.32 Degree of turbidity.

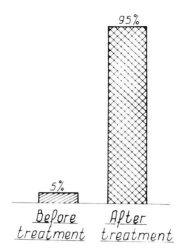

95%

5%

Before
treatment

After
treatment

Fig. 10.33 1st degree of turbidity.

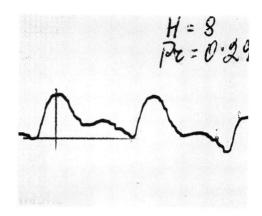

$H = 8$
$Pt = 0.29$

a

Consecutive application of IT and US

Authors who have applied ultrasound treatment in patients with Sudeck's atrophy stress that it results in reduction and relief of clinical symptoms without essentially influencing the X-ray findings. This is in line with some of our observations (Nikolova, 1979), i.e. that the X-ray image improves much more slowly. The more pronounced therapeutic effect of interferential therapy on X-ray findings can be explained by the stronger stimulation of metabolic processes and considerably improved microcirculation. As is well known, blood supply disorders in Sudeck's atrophy affect mainly the distal blood flow.

In a number of patients with Sudeck's atrophy, though typical changes disappeared or diminished after interferential therapy was applied, some residual phenomena such as slight pain and rigidity of joints due to e.g. poor reduction and free bone fragment were still observed. Ultrasound treatment in such patients is very helpful. This led us to study the consecutive application of IT and US to create a new multiple rehabilitation course.

Systematic observations were made on 50 patients (21 males and 29 females); 43 patients were aged between 31 and 60 and 7 patients were aged between 61 and 78. The basic causes for dystrophy, as shown by our other observations,

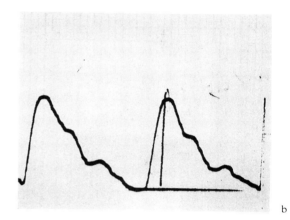

b

Fig. 10.34 Patient with post fractured right leg and 2nd stage Sudeck's atrophy. a. Before treatment, the rheographic curve is characterised by a round peak, lack of secondary waves and small amplitude, which is suggestive of increased arterial tone. b. After treatment with IC, there is a sharp rheographic peak, the presence of secondary waves and increased amplitude, which is indicative of decreased spasm and improved tissue blood supply.

were various bone fractures (42 patients) or some other injuries (8 patients). Wrong reduction was found in 20 patients. Fifteen patients were in the 1st stage of the disease, 29 in the 2nd stage and 6 in the 3rd stage.

Interferential current was applied first (see above), immediately followed by US within the dystrophy area using the labile technique for 6 to 12 minutes, at a dosage of 0.2–0.5 W/cm^2, for a total of 12 to 15 treatments.

The clinical symptoms and objective indices were favourably influenced from the 15th to the

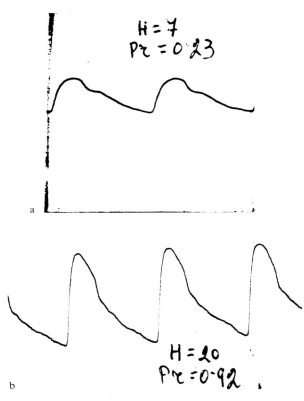

H = 7
Pr = 0·23

H = 20
Pr = 0·92

Fig. 10.35 Patient with post Colles' fracture and 2nd stage Sudeck's atrophy. a. Before treatment, there is a hypertonic rheographic curve with low amplitude, round peak and lack of sec waves. b. After IC treatment there is a normal rheographic curve with high amplitude, sharp peak and sec waves.

50th day on average depending on the start of the treatment and the concomitant complication (free bone fragment, etc.). Forty-two or 84% of patients were discharged with restored function, and 8 (16%) with elimination or relief of pain, improved movements and considerable reduction of trophic disturbances.

These data show that the final therapeutic results are somewhat better than when IT and US are applied separately. This can be accounted for by the mutual enhancement of the therapeutic effects. The vascular tone is regulated, interstitial oedema is more rapidly eliminated, the increased connective tissue is dispersed and muscle trophicity is improved.

Capillaroscopy before and after treatment was carried out in 20 patients with dystrophy of the upper extremity in the 2nd and 3rd stage. A reduced capillary count per visual field, spastically strictured shoulders of most capillary loops and grain-like blood flow were found. Marked improvement was noted after treatment, the capillaroscopic picture becoming the same or approaching that of the intact hand (Fig. 10.36). These changes were parallel to the clinical and X-ray findings. The control capillaroscopy in 2 patients with incomplete clinical recovery showed that the capillary loops were still spastic in their shoulders, the blood flow was grain-like and the halo preserved. Thus capillaroscopy in Sudeck's atrophy can be used to evaluate a method's therapeutic effect.

Calcitonin treatment was introduced in Sudeck's atrophy in 1973, and a number of authors reported that it had a beneficial effect, especially in the 1st and 2nd stage of the disease. According to the latest investigations (Portias, 1977), however, the drug's effectiveness is not apparent in clinical or X-ray examinations. As far as drug therapy is concerned, it should be pointed out that different authors have recommended a variety of medicines. Having traced many of the proposed and applied medicines (bamethan sulphate, kallidnogenase, nicotinyl alcohol), Wagner, one of the most outstanding specialists in Sudeck's atrophy, claimed that the evolution of atrophy without these drugs was neither more severe nor longer than when they were administered (Wagner, 1960). Our observations have shown that IT, when combined with appropriate drugs (nicotinyl alcohol, bamethan sulphate), will undoubtedly promote healing, especially in faulty reduction.

The following examples illustrate the marked therapeutic effect of interferential therapy separately or in conjunction with ultrasound:

A 48-year-old patient was in a car accident on June 26th, 1975. He had a severe longitudinal thrust on the right leg and contusion of the head, resulting in pain and moderate oedema in the knee joint. He did not see a doctor. His state deteriorated, the right lower extremity could not take weight and movements became difficult and painful. About 3 months later an orthopaedist diagnosed a torn meniscus and a meniscectomy was performed on September 21st, 1975.

The patient stayed in hospital for 1 month without purposeful rehabilitation. Later, remedial exercises were undertaken in combination with diadynamic current and ultrasound, but his condition continued to deteriorate.

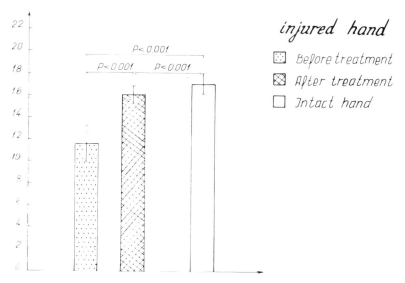

Fig. 10.36 Capillaries' count in 2nd stage Sudeck's atrophy.

Seven months after the injury, 4 months after the operation, he was sent to the Institute of Orthopaedics and Traumatology in Sofia. Electrophoresis treatment with Novocain was provided, which also turned out to be ineffective. Only then was he referred to our Clinic with a diagnosis of post meniscectomy, 3rd stage Sudeck's atrophy of the right patella, tibia and foot. The right knee joint and foot were oedematous, the musculature round the knee was hypotrophic, function of the knee and ankle joints was increasingly restricted and the patient walked with a stick. The X-ray showed a strongly marked algodystrophy of the knee joint, clearly visible coarse lacunar dystrophy of the patella (Fig. 10.37a) and milder but similar changes in the tibia and femur. A traumatic dystrophic cyst in the central axis of the head of the tibia was noticed.

After treatment with IT and ultrasound, the pain disappeared, function of the joint was restored and the X-ray appearance was normalised (Fig. 10.37b). Even the traumatic dystrophic cyst disappeared. The bony framework — longitudinal and transverse — was restored both in the patella and the two large bones. The same applied to the bones of the foot (Fig. 10.38b).

A 51-year-old patient had an accident on January 9th, 1977 and sustained a fracture of the forearm. Plaster immobilisation for 39 days was followed by warm baths and massage. Her condition deteriorated and she was sent for rehabilitation to our Clinic on July 10th, 1977 (6 months after the fracture) with a diagnosis of old right Colles' fracture with avulsion of the ulnar styloid, 2nd-3rd stage Sudeck's atrophy and contracture of the elbow joint (Fig. 10.39). As shown in Figure 10.39a, osteoporosis affected not only the epiphyseal areas of the carpal and phalangeal bones but also those of the radiocarpal bones with severe involvement of the spongy structure of the small bones and the epiphysis of the radius. The contours of small carpal bones nearly disappeared.

Interferential therapy was alternated with US, result-

ing in restoration of function of the forearm (Fig. 10.40), and changes due to spotty osteoporosis were removed (Fig. 10.39b).

The results gained with IT, applied separately or alternated with US, have given us grounds to consider it a successful therapy for Sudeck's atrophy.

Osteomyelitis and periostitis

Physiotherapy for traumatic osteomyelitis is applied in the chronic stage using short wave, microwaves, ultraviolet irradiations and electrophoresis with zinc.

Interferential therapy in the treatment of traumatic chronic osteomyelitis was introduced by us (Nikolova, 1969e, 1971a). The same methods were applied as in delayed callus formation and Sudeck's atrophy. Good results are also obtained in treating periostitis. The electrodes for superficial action are used and the necessary 20 to 25 treatments are carried out daily for 15 minutes.

Osteochondropathy

The aetiology of osteochondropathy has not yet been completely elucidated, and so far the problem of its treatment has not been solved either. Interferential therapy in the treatment of

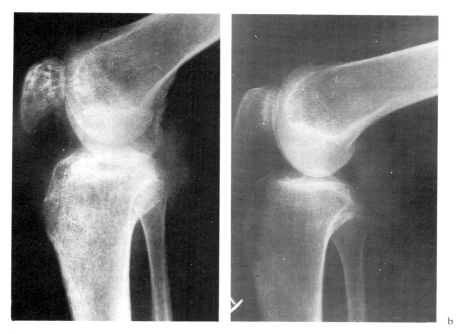

Fig. 10.37 X-ray of the right knee joint of a patient with 3rd stage Sudeck's atrophy, post meniscectomy. a. Before treatment, there is strongly pronounced before treatment.
b. X-ray after IC treatment — the calcium deposits are dispersed.

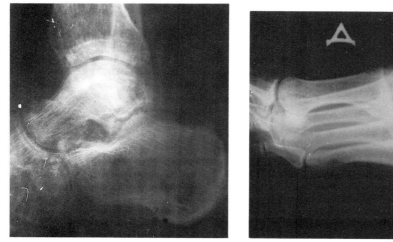
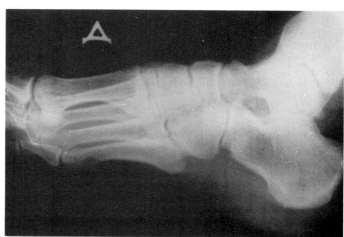

Fig. 10.38 Same patient as in Figure 10.37. a. X-ray before treatment showing Sudeck's atrophy of the foot. b. X-ray after treatment, showing normalisation of the X-ray image after IT.

osteochondropathy was first introduced in Bulgaria by us (Nikolova, 1969c). Having in mind the theory that aseptic necrosis develops in disturbed blood circulation in the affected areas, we applied interferential current at a constant frequency of 100 Hz and a rhythmical frequency of 90–100 Hz, since these two frequencies possess marked vasodilating and analgesic effects.

Treatment is applied with 4-plate (or vacuum) electrodes which, depending on the type of

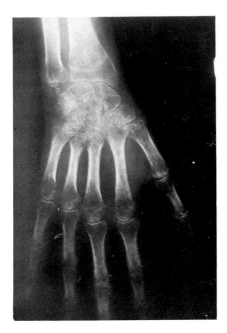

a

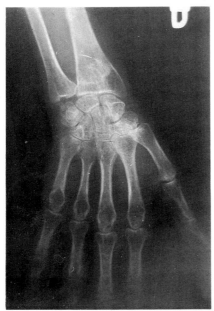

b

Fig. 10.39 Patient with 2nd-3rd stage Sudeck's atrophy.
a. X-ray before treatment with IC and US. b. X-ray after
treatment, showing normalisation of the bone structure.

osteochondropathy being treated, are positioned
in such a manner that the involved area is in the
interference zone. Twenty treatments are given
daily for 15 to 20 minutes. After a 10-day break,

therapy is repeated and if necessary it is applied
for the third time.

A total of 110 patients with osteochondropathies at different sites were observed by us (Table
10.8). The disease process was favourably influenced, pain diminished or disappeared, oedema
dispersed and normal movements were restored
in all but 1 patient. Control X-rays were taken in
60 patients with osteochondropathy and in all
patients with avascular necrosis. They revealed
recovery of bone structure in all patients with
avascular necrosis and in 32 patients with osteochondropathy.

The oscillographic and rheographic examinations showed the following:

1. Before treatment there was asymmetry
    with a lowered oscillographic and rheogra-
    phic index in the affected limb in 75% of
    the patients. This is to be expected in view
    of the disturbed arterial blood circulation
    in osteochondropathy.
2. After completion of treatment there was an
    absence of asymmetry or a tendency for
    asymmetry to be smoothed in the oscillo-
    graphic and rheographic index in 80% of
    the investigated patients. This is an indica-
    tion of stable improvement of blood irriga-
    tion due to IT.

It should be stressed that we were not able to
find reports in the available medical literature
with X-ray evidence of the beneficial effect of
other physiotherapeutic methods on aseptic necrosis. For that reason we consider that our
observations on the positive effect of IC in
aseptic necrosis are very important.

Styloiditis and epicondylitis

Epicondylitis and styloiditis are noted by Nemec
(1966) as being treatable by interferential current.
No data are available, however, on the clinical
results. We have applied treatment to 50 patients
(40 with epicondylitis and 10 with styloiditis),
aged between 20 and 60, 34 women and 16 men
(obviously the number of women is predominant). The therapy was provided with 4-plate
electrodes or a 4-field electrode (Fig. 10.41a), and
also with tetra-polar vacuum electrodes using the

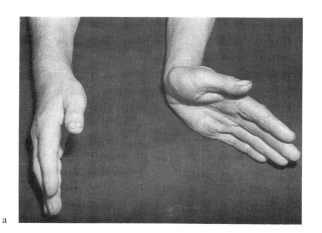

a

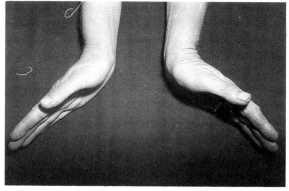

d

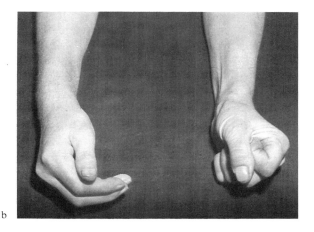

b

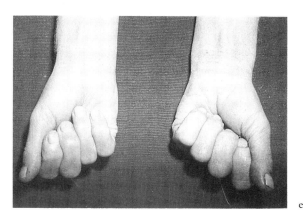

e

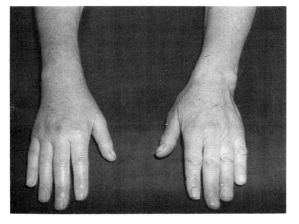

c

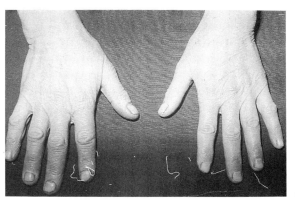

f

Fig. 10.40 Same patient as in Figure 10.39. a,b,c. Functional condition before IC and US treatment. d,e,f. Functional repair after treatment.

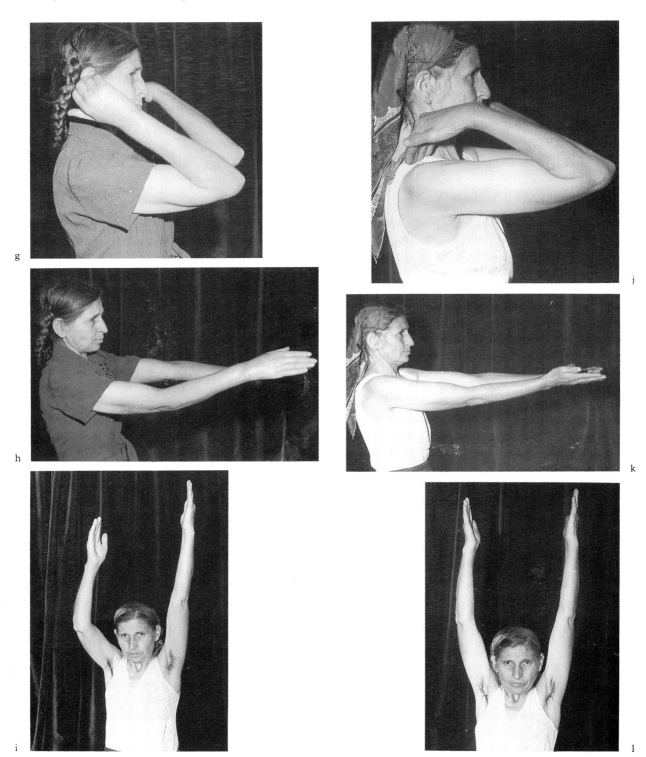

Fig. 10.40 (contd.) g,h,i. Functional condition before IC and US treatment. j,k,l. Functional repair after treatment.

Table 10.8 Distribution of site of osteochondropathies

Site	Number of patients
Tuberosity of tibia (Osgood-Schlatter)	35
Lunate bone (Kienboeck)	10
Tarsal navicular bone (Koehler)	5
Upper femoral epiphysis (Perthes)	25
Calcaneum (Schinz)	10
Traumatic avascular necrosis	25

a

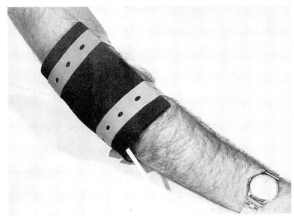

b

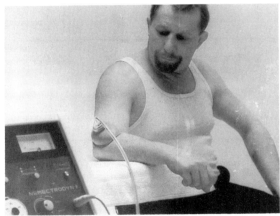

Fig. 10.41 Position of electrodes in treating epicondylitis. a. With a 4-field electrode. b. With a vacuum electrode.

Nemectrodyn-8 apparatus (Fig. 10.41b). The first 3 treatments were applied at a constant frequency of 100 Hz, and the remaining at a frequency of 0–100 Hz.[16] A total of 10 to 20 procedures were given daily for 15 minutes (Nikolova, 1971a).

[16] Good results using IT were reported later by Eigler (1980).

Very good results were obtained when interferential therapy was alternated with ultrasound or microwaves.

The following example illustrates the beneficial therapeutic results of IT:

> A 45-year-old patient felt a mild pain in the outer side of the left elbow joint irradiating to the dorsal side of the forearm. She was treated with intra-articular hydrocortisone and with diadynamic current. The complaints were significantly relieved. Later on, after 2 to 3 months, she again felt a violent pain after work related to physical strain of the left hand, and movements were restricted. The arm was put in a splint for 25 days. Ultrasound treatment failed. An operation was suggested — decortication of the radial epicondyle — but the patient refused.
>
> She was admitted to our Clinic with a diagnosis of right humeral epicondylitis, tenovaginitis of the forearm and contracture of the elbow following immobilisation. Interferential therapy resulted in removal of subjective complaints and restoration of movements of the elbow joint (Fig. 10.42).

CONDITIONS OF MUSCLES, TENDONS, AND BURSAE

Myalgia

The positive effect of interferential current in treating myalgia has been established by many authors (Burghart, 1952; Nikolova, 1971a; Ganne, 1976).

Treatment is provided with 4-plate, 4-field or 2-field electrodes, and also as interferential electrokinesy with glove electrodes. A current of a constant frequency of 100 Hz is applied during the first 3 treatments followed by a current of a rhythmical frequency of 0–100 Hz over a period of 10 to 15 minutes. Complaints usually subside after 2 to 10 procedures. A combination with vacuum massage is recommended especially when there is pain in the lumbosacral region. Interferential electrokinesy gives excellent results in myalgia nuchae.

Myositis

Interferential therapy in treating myositis of infectious, toxic or traumatic aetiology is used in the following two ways: (1) in combination with vacuum massage or vibromassage (Vibrodyn apparatus); (2) with glove electrodes at a rhythmical frequency of 0–100 Hz. The necessary 10 to

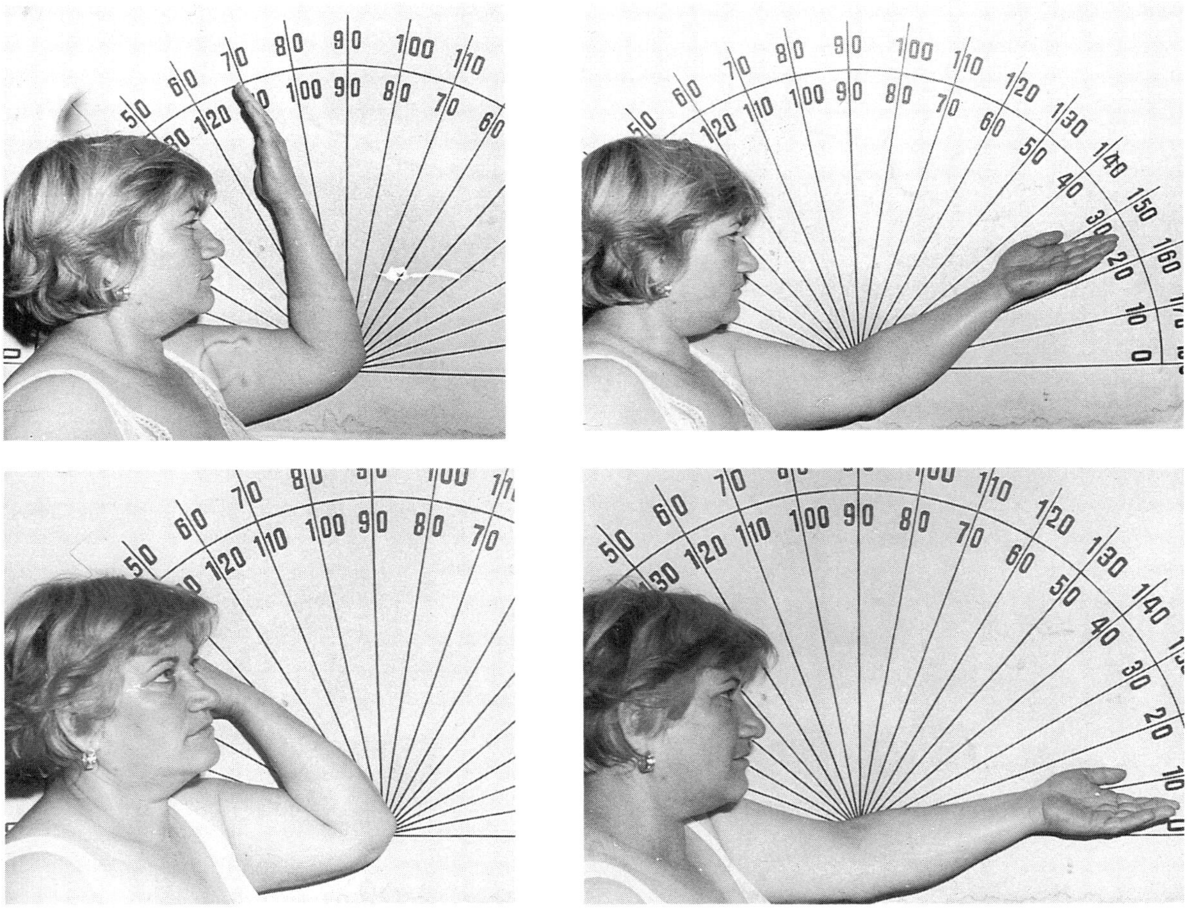

Fig. 10.42 Patient with extension-flexion contracture of the elbow joint secondary to immobilisation. a,b. Before treatment. c,d. After IC treatment.

15 treatments are applied for 10 to 12 minutes daily.

Myositis ossificans

Knowing the considerable difficulties of treating myositis ossificans, we started to apply IC in this condition in 1964. We had good reason to select this type of electrotherapy, since IC at a rhythmical frequency of 0–100 Hz, as has been noted before, has analgesic effects, activates metabolic processes, improves tissue trophicity and assists the active elimination of haematomata and adhesions.

The electrodes are placed in such a manner that the area of myositis is exactly within the area of the beat frequency. The current intensity depends on the area of the electrodes and the individual tolerance of the patient, who should experience the usual slight tingling sensation. The patient attends daily for 15 minutes; a total of 20 treatments constitute a therapeutic course. It is advisable to combine IT with remedial exercises consisting of gentle, painless active movements.

We observed 40 patients aged between 6 and 50 with myositis ossificans. The condition was observed in the shoulder in 3 patients, in the elbow joint in 25 and the remaining patients had the condition in various areas of the lower extremities. In 15 patients the condition developed after injuries such as bruising, sprain or dislocation, and in the others following fractures.

Thermotherapy such as paraffin wax applications or hot baths had been applied in 32 patients (80%), and additionally also passive movements with massage, weight-lifting and hanging from hands in 20 patients (50%). These data were suggestive of the basic cause of the disease — wrong methods of treatment.

Therapeutic results using IT were assessed with the following measuring devices: tape measure, goniometer and X-ray. Beneficial effects were observed in 36 patients. In 14 of them myositis was not revealed on the radiographs.

The results gained indicate great progress in the medical treatment of myositis ossificans due to IC. The belief of some authors that the use of physiotherapy for treating myositis ossificans is contraindicated is thus disproved. Only unsuitable, incorrect physiotherapy (forced movements, massage, hot baths) can be considered to be contraindicated. We think that surgical treatment in myositis ossificans should not be applied before the therapeutic effect of IC at a rhythmical frequency of 0–100 Hz has been tried.

Volkmann's ischaemic muscle contracture

In treating this condition it is important first to eliminate the factors which have led to disturbances of blood circulation, and then methods should be applied which help to do away with the vascular-dystrophic process. Interferential current was introduced by us in 1963 in the treatment of the disease, since at a constant frequency of 100 Hz it has a marked vasodilating and analgesic effect. The whole arm is included in the field (Fig. 7.6) or alternatively the thoracic ganglion, daily for 15, 20 or 25 minutes, with a total of 15 to 20 treatments in a therapeutic course.

Ruptured muscle fibres

Interferential therapy in the treatment of muscle ruptures gives very good results, since it not only relieves pain and leads to resorption of the haematomata, but also accelerates the repair of muscle fibres. It is applied with 4-plate electrodes, positioned so that the ruptured region is in the centre of the field. A rhythmical frequency of 0–100 Hz is used daily for 5, 10 or 15 minutes until complete restoration of function is reached. Interferential electrokinesy is used when the condition has been present for a long time. Stimulation is given proximally and distally to the area of the rupture.

Ruptured tendons

Surgical treatment to suture the tendons is the first priority. After immobilisation we recommend IT at a rhythmical frequency of 0–100 Hz for 15 minutes daily (Nikolova, 1971a) to restore function. It contributes to relieving pain, oedema and trophic disorders, and therefore a more rapid restoration of function is obtained.

Interferential current also gives good results in the treatment of teno-periosteal inflammation (inflammation of the elbow flexor insertions due to overwork), according to our observations of more than 50 patients. It is conducted at a rhythmical frequency of 0–100 Hz or a constant frequency of 100 Hz if accompanied by strong pain during the first few days. The following example illustrates the beneficial effect of IT:

> A 54-year-old concrete worker fell ill on September 2nd, 1966 with violent pains in the right elbow joint and swelling of the arm. He was treated with drugs, fomentations and ultratherm but his condition deteriorated. The patient was referred to us on September 29th, 1966 with a diagnosis of teno-periosteal inflammation with contracture of the elbow joint. On admission, he had pain and constriction in the right elbow joint, the pain being violent in the area of insertion of the biceps muscle, and a flexion contracture of 40°. The blood picture and erythrocyte sedimentation rate were normal. Symmetrical radiographs of the two elbow joints showed very slight changes in the soft tissues of the right joint — periostosis in the volar aspect of the olecranon and capsular calcification of the elbow joint. After establishing a diagnosis of inflammation at the insertion of the brachioradialis muscle, interferential therapy was applied at a rhythmical frequency of 0–100 and 0–10 Hz (alternated every other day), for a total of 15 treatments. Flexion contracture was repressed and the function of the arm was restored. The patient was able to resume work.

Scapulohumeral periarthritis

In spite of numerous investigations, the aetiology of periarthritis of the shoulder joint is not yet fully understood. Acute or chronic trauma (the importance of major trauma is acknowledged by all authors) is considered to be the most common cause, followed by other causes such as previous infection, metabolic disorders or exposure to cold (e.g. drivers who leave the window open in cold weather).

No unanimous opinion is available concerning suitable therapeutic management of this disease. Various drugs, Novocain blocks and intra-articular injections with hydrocortisone are recommended. The importance of physiotherapy is recognised by all authors, but they disagree on the method of choice. Interferential therapy in this condition has been applied by us since October 1963. Only the report of Paleirah et al (1956) was found in the literature at that time. He had successfully applied this method in four patients only.

We provided out-patient therapy to all patients using the following methods: 4-plate electrodes of an area of 50 or 100 cm^2 each (or vacuum electrodes) were placed above and below the affected joint in such a manner that the joint should be in the interference area (Fig. 7.7), which is very important for the therapeutic effect. Treatments were applied daily with a current of a constant frequency of 100 Hz for the first 3 days, followed by a rhythmical frequency of 0–100 Hz, for 15 minutes, for a total of 20 procedures. The current intensity is 12–25 mA, depending on the area of the electrodes and the patient's individual tolerance, who should experience a strong but pleasant tingling sensation — a sensation of pleasant massage in depth. Often, even after only 1 to 3 treatments, pain is relieved and movements are improved.

The choice of the above frequencies is made because of the analgesic property and the suppressive effect on the sympathetic system at the first frequency. The second frequency leads to active hyperaemia, improves the metabolic processes and rapidly eliminates toxic products and restores normal tissue reactions.

Interferential current only was applied in 320 patients between 1963 and 1970; IC combined with microwaves (alternating every other day) was used in 130 patients. The effect of these methods was compared to that of microwaves, ultrasound, diadynamic current and radiotherapy (Table 10.9). A total of 450 patients (184 males and 266 females) were treated with IC only, or with IC combined with microwaves. The age distribution of the patients was as follows: 15 patients were aged between 20 and 30 years; 310 were aged between 31 and 50; 90 were aged between 51 and 60 and 35 were aged between 61 and 70. These data show the highest incidence between the ages of 30 and 60, i.e. the most actively working population (Nikolova, 1966b, 1970d,e). Therefore, prompt and efficient therapy is important not only from a humane but also from an economic point of view.

All the patients were admitted in the acute stage of the disease with severe pain, restricted or absent movement in the affected joint and pain on palpation in the greater tuberosity area. Initial X-rays showed calcium deposits of different sizes in 416 patients. Concomitant osteoarthrosis of the shoulder joint was found in 82 patients and cervical arthrosis in 56 patients.

Table 10.9 Comparison of IT and other methods in treating scapulohumeral periarthritis

Applied therapeutic methods	Number of patients	Therapeutic results*			
		Healthy	Greatly improved	Improved	No effect
IC	320	240(75%)	42(13%)	32(10%)	6(2%)
IC and microwaves	130	104(80%)	21(16%)	5(4%)	–
Microwaves	100	38(38%)	46(46%)	10(10%)	6(6%)
Diadynamic current	35	10(29%)	12(34%)	11(31%)	2(6%)
Ultrasound	70	13(19%)	27(39%)	17(24%)	13(18%)
Radiotherapy	60	9(15%)	9(15%)	8(13%)	34(57%)

* 'Healthy' = patients without subjective complaints and with a normal range of movements. 'Greatly improved' = patients discharged without pain at rest but with pain occurring at certain times and from certain movements. 'Improved' = patients with incomplete restoration of normal movement because of mild pain

Interferential therapy proved to be the most effective treatment, as was shown by our investigation of a total of 715 patients (Table 10.9) (Nikolova, 1966b, 1970d,e). The highest percentage of patients without response had received radiotherapy.[17] In addition, the control radiographs in 250 patients enabled us to find out another new property of IC, i.e. the ability to disperse pathological calcium deposits at a rhythmical frequency of 0–100 Hz (Figs 10.43 and 10.44). Complete dispersion was established in 40% of the patients,[18] partial in 30% and the X-ray findings remained unchanged in 30%. As shown by our observations, deposits are more rapidly and easily dispersed in patients with a shorter history of the condition. There is not a complete correspondence, however, between dispersion of calcium deposits and clinical recovery.[19] Recovery of function is also more rapid in recent cases. Therefore IT should be employed as early as possible.

Long-term results were traced in 100 patients. Recurrence after 4 to 8 months was encountered in 7 patients, and after 1 to 4 years in 23. Function was eventually restored in these patients also after repeated interferential therapy. The excellent results obtained from IT are illustrated by the following examples:

For 3 to 4 years this patient had complained of dull pain in the right shoulder joint on sudden movements. She had not been given any treatment. On August 22nd, 1976 after over-fatigue, she felt severe pain in the shoulder with completely restricted movements. Analgesic drugs proved ineffective, and she was admitted for treatment with a diagnosis of acute scapulohumeral periarthritis (Fig. 10.45). In addition to the severe pain, there was no movement in the right shoulder joint (Fig. 10.46a,b,c). Sixteen IC treatments were applied, resulting in dispersion of the calcium deposit (Fig. 10.45b), relief of pain and complete restoration of function (Fig. 10.46d,e,f). Long-term results were reviewed for a 6-year period, and it was found that the patient had no complaints.

[17] When radiotherapy has failed to produce an effect (or has aggravated the patient's condition) IT can be applied successfully with no side effects.

[18] Pathological calcium deposits can also be observed in the area of other joints and are also dispersed by interferential therapy.

[19] As soon as the pain subsided remedial exercises were also included in the treatment. IC combined with ultrasound was applied mainly in patients with long-standing calcium deposits; IC with microwaves was used in

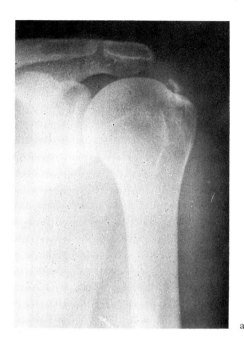

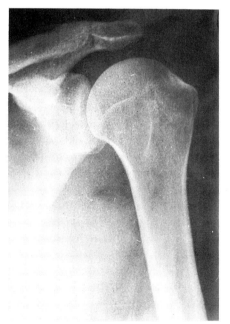

Fig. 10.43 Patient with periarthritis of the left shoulder joint. a. X-ray before treatment. b. X-ray after IT, showing dispersion of calcium deposits.

concomitant deforming arthrosis. Local treatment was applied in all patients with cervical arthrosis together with ultrasound or with glove electrodes in the relevant paravertebral area.

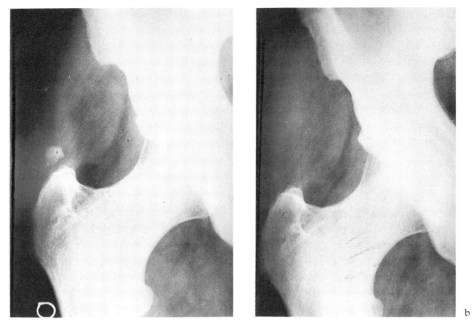

a

b

Fig. 10.44 Patient with periarthritis of the right hip joint. a. X-ray before treatment. b. X-ray after IC treatment — the calcium deposits are dispersed.

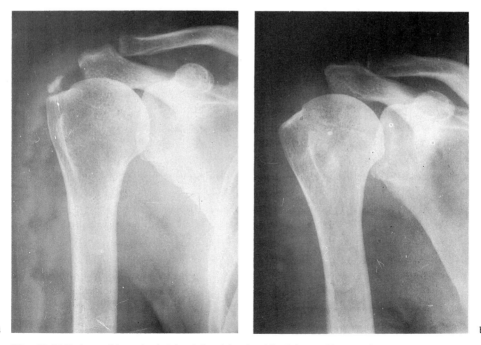

a

b

Fig. 10.45 Patient with periarthritis of the right shoulder joint. a. X-ray before treatment. b. X-ray after IC treatment — the calcium deposits are dispersed.

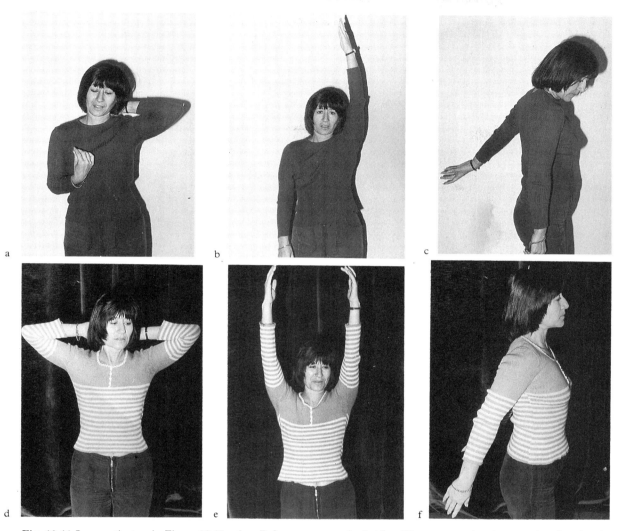

Fig. 10.46 Same patient as in Figure 10.45. a,b,c. Before treatment. d,e,f. After IC treatment, showing complete functional repair.

A 53-year-old hospital attendant woke on September 4th, 1977 with severe pain in the left shoulder joint and was unable to look after herself. On September 5th, 1977 she was examined by an orthopaedist. X-rays showed calcium deposits in the area of the greater tuberosity. The patient was immediately referred to our Clinic with a diagnosis of acute left-sided scapulohumeral periarthritis. A total of 15 IT treatments were applied, resulting in dispersion of calcium deposits, relief of pain and complete restoration of function (Fig. 10.47).

The effect of IT, US and magnetotherapy in periarthritis with calcium deposits

Ultrasound, phonophoresis with hydrocortisone paste or phenylbutazone emulsion has been used for a long time in patients with periarthritis of the shoulder joint. There are a number of reports on the beneficial therapeutic effect of magnetotherapy, which is accounted for by the pain-relieving, antiphlogistic and trophic action of the low-frequency magnetic field. These authors, however, have not compared their therapeutic results with those obtained from other physiotherapeutic methods. It has also been reported that the consecutive application (one immediately after the other) of IC and ultrasound enhances their therapeutic effect. We were thus prompted to compare the effects of (1) IT alone, (2) the

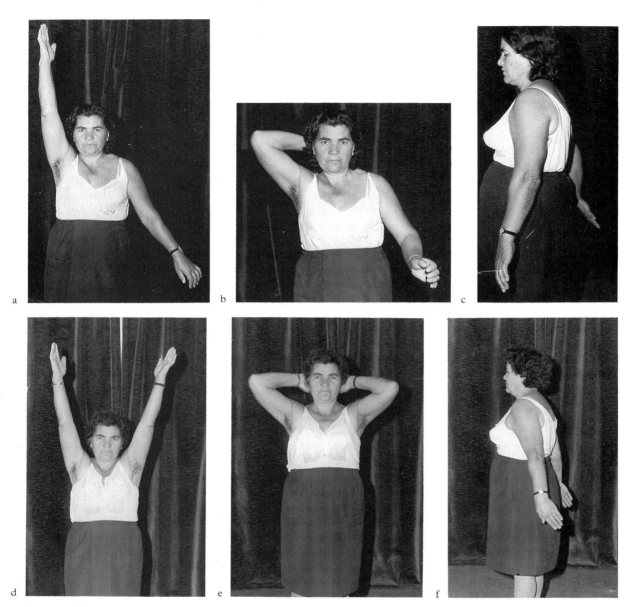

Fig. 10.47 Patient with periarthritis of the left shoulder joint. a,b,c. Before treatment. d,e,f. After IC treatment (15 procedures), showing complete functional restoration.

consecutive application of IT and US and (3) magnetotherapy alone.

We applied IT and US in the following way: IT given first, immediately followed by US in the shoulder joint area at a dosage of 0.2–0.6 W/cm² over a period of 8 to 12 minutes, for a total of 10, 12 or 15 treatments. Magnetotherapy was carried out in a continuous field, the affected joints being

placed between the two inductors closely applied to the skin. Procedures were carried out daily at a dosage of 40–50 mT over a period of 10 to 15 minutes, for a total of 15 to 20 procedures.

Our observations covered a total of 120 patients: 51 men and 69 women. Twenty-two patients were up to 40 years old; 86 were aged between 41 and 60 and 12 were over 60. In 42 patients the aetiology was found to be an acute or chronic trauma, and in 78 it was physical overfatigue. The duration of the condition was as follows: 65 patients had had symptoms for 10 to 30 days, 33 patients for 3 to 4 months, 19 patients for 2 to 4 years and 3 patients for over 10 years. All the patients were admitted in the acute stage with severe shooting pains, restricted movements or complete inability to move the shoulder joint, pain on palpation of the greater tuberosity, night pain disturbing sleep and incapacity for work. Calcium deposits of different sizes were found in

104 patients. The results of the comparative studies are presented in Table 10.10 and Figure 10.48.

Restoration of function occurred earlier in consecutive application of IT and US (12 to 15 days on average) than if the two methods were applied separately, which suggests that they mutually enhance their therapeutic effects. Dispersion of calcium deposits was established in the three methods without any statistically significant differences ($p > 0.05$). Restoration of flexion using the first two methods is of greater statistical

Table 10.10 Comparison of IT, IT and US and magnetotherapy in treating periarthritis of the shoulder joint

Applied therapeutic method	Number of patients	Therapeutic results*		
		Healthy	Various degrees of improvement	No effect
IT	30	21(70%)	9(30%)	–
IT and US applied consecutively	60	48(80%)	12(20%)	–
Magnetotherapy	30	14(47%)	10(33%)	6(20%)

* 'Healthy' = no complaints, with normal extent of movements. 'Various degrees of improvement' = no spontaneous pains; pains occur at a definite extent of movement

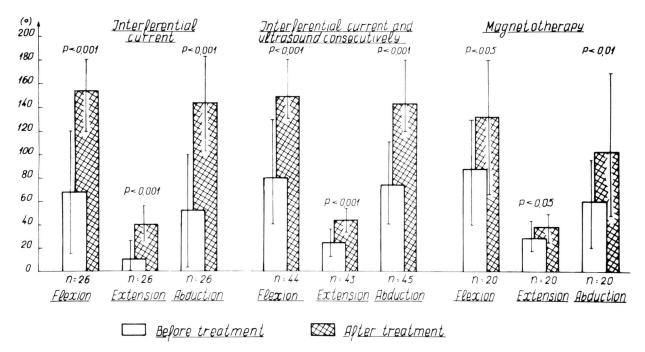

Fig. 10.48 Summary of the therapeutic results in treating periarthritis with calcium deposits.

significance (p < 0.001) than in magnetotherapy (p < 0.01). Six of the patients were not influenced by magnetotherapy.

The biochemical indices (sodium, potassium, chlorine, phosphorus) were within the norm before and after treatment with statistically insignificant changes after therapy for each index (p > 0.05).

The results obtained are illustrated by the following examples:

A 52-year-old patient had pain in the left shoulder joint for 2 months, which became intolerable in spite of analgesic drugs. Movements were painful and restricted. An X-ray showed massive calcium deposits, and a diagnosis of left scapulohumeral periarthritis and cervical arthrosis was established. After 15 treatments with IC and US, calcium deposits were dispersed, pain disappeared and function was restored (Fig. 10.49).

A 43-year-old patient slipped, fell and struck her right shoulder joint on December 25th, 1978. She had severe pain. A week later she went to see a traumatologist. An X-ray showed massive calcium deposits. Treatment was given with indomethacin, phonophoresis with hydrocortisone and short wave, for a total of 7 procedures. Treatment was interrupted because she left for the country. Later on she had rather severe pain and could not move her hand. She was admitted to our Clinic on February 16th, 1979 with a diagnosis of right scapulohumeral periarthritis. The pain that she had had for 3 to 4 days was strong both at rest and when she tried to do certain movements. The joint was blocked and she was not able to look after herself (Fig. 10.50a,b).

Interferential therapy alternated with ultrasound was given resulting in dispersion of calcium deposits, relief of pain and complete restoration of function (Fig. 10.50c,d).

A 42-year-old fitter had suffered from violent pain in the left shoulder both at rest and on movement since November 5th, 1976. He had been given drugs, but the pain persisted and became intolerable, particularly at night. Movements of the shoulder were impossible. The patient was admitted for hospital treatment, which included diadynamic current, iontophoresis, ultraviolet irradiation and underwater exercises resulting in slight improvement only. An X-ray showed a massive calcium deposit. He was sent to our Clinic with a diagnosis of left scapulohumeral periarthritis. Pain was severe and active and passive movements in the shoulder were restricted. Interferential therapy alternated with ultrasound led to dispersion of calcium deposits, relief of pain and restoration of arm function (Fig. 10.51).

A 49-year-old patient fell ill suddenly at the beginning of March 1979. An X-ray taken on March 6th showed calcium deposits in the area of the left shoulder joint. The patient was referred to our Clinic with severe pain and restricted movement in the shoulder joint. Interferential therapy (23 procedures) alternating with US (15 procedures) resulted in dispersion of calcium deposits, relief of pain and restoration of movements in the affected joint (Fig. 10.52).

Analysis of the results in the three groups of patients showed they were nearly the same

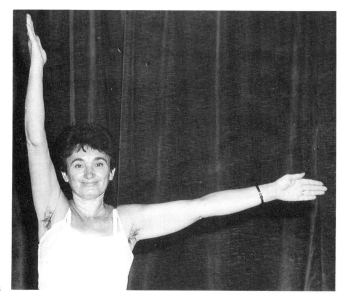
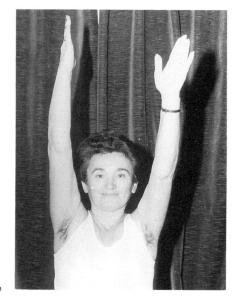

Fig. 10.49 Patient with left scapulohumeral periarthritis and cervical arthritis. a. Before treatment with IC and US. b. After IT, showing complete repair of function.

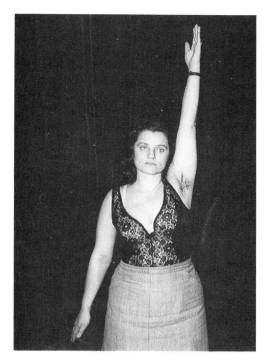

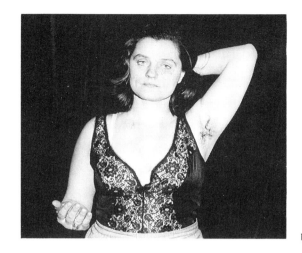

a

b

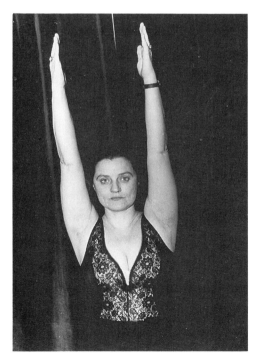

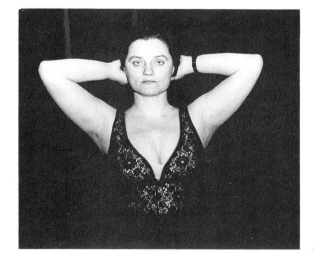

c

d

Fig. 10.50 Patient with right scapulohumeral periarthritis. a,b. Before treatment with IC and US. c,d. After IT, showing repair of function.

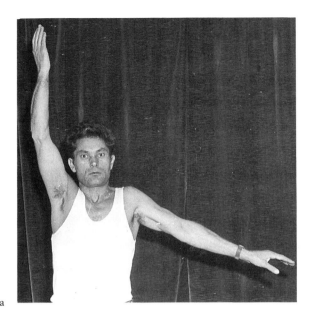

a

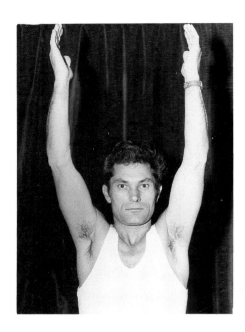

b

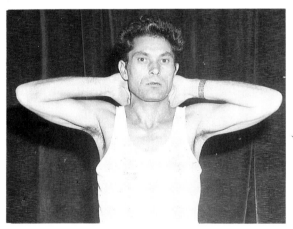

c

Fig. 10.51 Patient with left scapulohumeral periarthritis. a. Before treatment with IC and US. b,c. After treatment, showing repair of function.

netic field is statistically insignificant ($p > 0.05$). Magnetotherapy requires a higher number of treatments to attain restoration of function, with recurrence being more common.

The following practical conclusions can be drawn:

1. Interferential therapy gives better results than any other method under study.
2. Interferential therapy alternated with ultrasound has limited application and is not a universal method of pain relief in other conditions of the shoulder, such as tuberculosis and malignant neoplasms.
3. The therapeutic effect of magnetotherapy is less beneficial than IT alternated with ultrasound, as far as the immediate results and the lasting therapeutic effect are concerned.

'Frozen shoulder'

Scapulohumeral periarthritis is sometimes difficult to differentiate from so-called 'frozen shoulder' (adhesive capsulitis). 'Frozen shoulder' is a manifestation of a chronic adhesive process of the synovia where the latter shrinks greatly and sticks to the humeral head. No X-ray changes are found. Clinically, shoulder movements are re-

($p < 0.05$) in the first and second group, while in the magnetotherapy group there is a statistically significant difference ($p < 0.001$). Restoration of flexion, extension and abduction in the shoulder joint after treatment is statistically significant in the three groups, especially with the first two methods (Table 10.10 and Fig. 10.48). Dispersion of calcium deposits is more pronounced in the first two groups, but the difference in comparison with patients treated with a low-frequency mag-

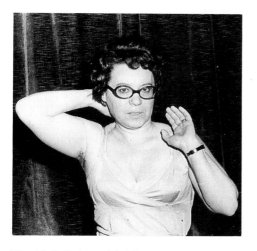
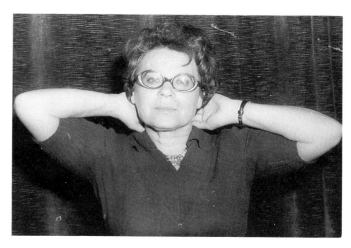

a   b

Fig. 10.52 Patient with left scapulohumeral periarthritis. a. Before IC and US treatment. b. After treatment, showing functional restoration.

stricted, especially the movements of external rotation and abduction. Various injuries in the shoulder area can be cited as aetiological factors. Pain appears first on movement and then becomes constant. Many authors feel that physiotherapeutic methods fail if the adhesions are not torn under anaesthesia.

Interferential therapy has a marked beneficial effect in treating 'frozen shoulder'. Two examples illustrate this point:

A 55-year-old accountant had dizziness during a hypertension crisis with equilibrium disturbance, making her stagger and strike her shoulder joint. At the moment of the blow she felt an acute, violent pain in the shoulder. She did not see a doctor. Twenty days later the pain became so severe that it 'paralysed' the shoulder and all movements. On examination in hospital a 'frozen shoulder' was diagnosed. Three betamethasone injections were given intra-articularly and 7 treatments of iontophoresis with Novocain. The therapy failed and her condition did not change.

She was referred to our Clinic with a diagnosis of 2nd degree hypertension and frozen shoulder of the left arm. Twenty-five treatments with IC were carried out (the first 3 at a constant frequency of 100 Hz, and the remaining at a rhythmical frequency of 0–100 Hz) resulting in gradual relief of pain followed by restoration of normal movements (Fig. 10.53).

In March 1978 a patient felt severe pain in the left shoulder joint. 'Brachial plexitis' was diagnosed on examination. Treatment with analgesics and vitamins was given. The pain increased and movements in the joint were restricted. The patient was treated with betamethasone injected intra-articularly. Pain diminished but joint restriction still persisted. She was examined in the Institute of Orthopaedics and Traumatology. 'Frozen

shoulder' was diagnosed and movements under anaesthesia were proposed. She refused and was referred to our Clinic about 6 months after the onset of the disease.

A total of 25 treatments with IC and 15 treatments with US were applied in conjunction with cautious remedial exercises after the pain subsided. As a result pain was relieved, the function of the hand was restored (Fig. 10.54) and the patient returned to work.

CONDITIONS OF JOINTS

Congenital dislocation of the hip (CDH)

Interferential therapy in treating CDH was first introduced by us in 1963. It is applied in the postoperative period.

Before removal of plaster

The purpose is to relieve pain and muscle spasm, stimulate callus formation in the osteotomy area (irrespective of internal fixation in some cases) and prevent postoperative complications.

Interferential therapy is carried out by cutting small apertures in the plaster. A current of a constant frequency of 100 Hz or a rhythmical frequency of 90–100 Hz is provided daily on the operated joint or the whole extremity for 15 to 20 minutes for a total of 12 to 20 treatments. The strength of the current is determined by the area of the electrodes so that the patient experiences mild, pleasant sensations.

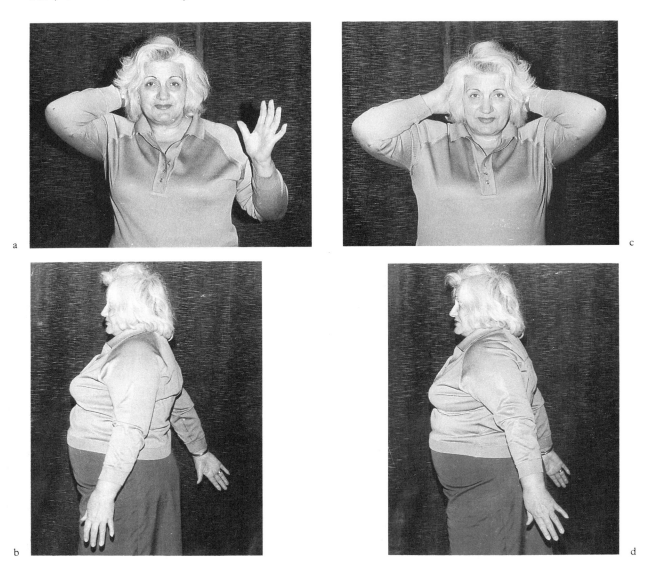

Fig. 10.53 Patient with left frozen shoulder. a,b. Before IC treatment. c,d. After IT, showing restoration of function.

The treatment can be combined with massage of those parts of the body which are free, as well as with remedial exercises and ultraviolet irradiation.

After removal of plaster

For the first few days the purpose is to eliminate muscle spasm in the operation area, to relieve pain and to regain the normal range of movement in the hip joint, as well as to prevent or reduce muscle atrophy and adaptive shortening.

Treatment is applied at a rhythmical frequency of 0–100 Hz (interference vector is preferable), acting separately on the hip and knee joints. The treatments are given one after the other daily or alternating every other day. At the same time, in addition to massage and remedial exercises, underwater jet massage and baths can be used.

Interferential therapy gives very good results in

these cases and should therefore become an integral part of the whole programme of rehabilitation.

Contusion

The subjective complaints of patients and pain on palpation and movement are conspicuous features in the clinical picture of bruised joints. In some cases the synovial sac reacts with an accumulation of serous fluid (synovial effusion) and, if the synovial membrane is disrupted, with haemarthrosis formation.

Treatment is conservative. A number of physiotherapeutic methods such as diadynamic cur-

rent and microwaves are applied more or less successfully. Interferential therapy is acknowledged to have a beneficial effect by all authors who have used it (Nikolova, 1966c, 1967b, 1971a, Fiedler, 1960 and others).

We have applied IC in 60 patients with contusion without haemarthrosis and in 20 with haemarthrosis. Interferential current of a rhythmical frequency of 90–100 Hz was used in the first 2 treatments, followed by a frequency of 0–100 Hz using the same method as in sprains. Treatment can be started as early as the first hours after the injury (in haemarthrosis, on the second day after aspiration). Complaints usually disappear even after the 2nd to the 5th treatment,

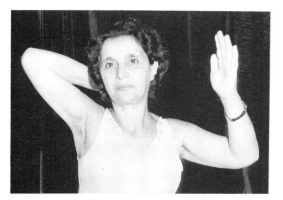
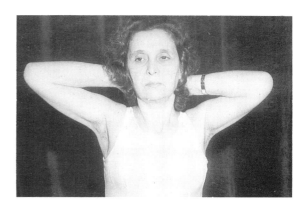
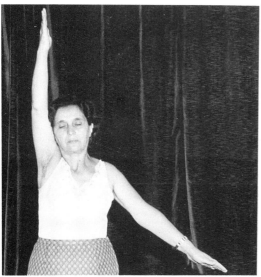
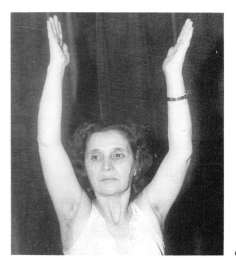

Fig. 10.54 Patient with left frozen shoulder. a,b. Before IC and US treatment. c,d. After treatment, showing functional repair.

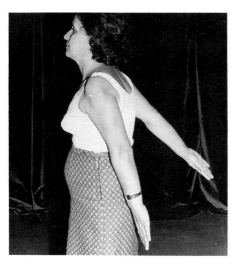

e

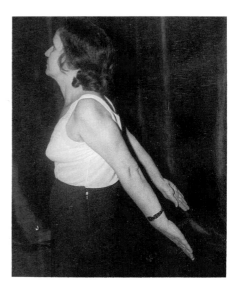

f

Fig. 10.54 (contd.) e. Before IC and US treatment. f. After treatment, showing functional restoration.

if treatment has begun in time. With effusions in particular the combination of IT with microwaves has given excellent results, and compared with other physiotherapeutic methods IC has been proved to be the most effective (Table 10.11).

To illustrate the excellent results of IT, two examples are given:

> A 23-year-old fitter slipped, fell and struck his left elbow joint on January 25th, 1981, resulting in pain, oedema and painful and restricted movements. An X-ray did not show any fracture. A soft compression bandage was applied and analgesics were prescribed. Swelling increased in the next few days, pain became more severe and movements were impossible. After a check-up on

> February 5th, 1981, sick-leave was continued and microwaves and remedial exercises were given. Because this treatment failed, another traumatologist was consulted. Eventually the patient was referred to our Clinic a month after the injury with permanent flexion-extension contracture (Fig. 10.55a,b). Interferential therapy was provided, resulting in restoration of function (Fig. 10.55c,d) in 20 'days' time, after which the patient returned to his work.

> A 39-year-old patient had a condition dating back 3 months when she had struck her right elbow joint against a hard object. The pain gradually increased, and movements in the elbow joint were restricted.

> She was admitted to our Clinic with a diagnosis of periarthritis with calcification and stiffening of the right elbow following a blow. Interferential current and

Table 10.11 Comparison of IT and other methods in treating contusion of joints

Applied therapeutic method	Number of patients	Therapeutic results*		
		Healthy	Different degrees of improvement	No effect
IC	80	60(75%)	20(25%)	–
IC and microwaves	10	10(100%)	–	–
Diadynamic current	35	18(51%)	15(43%)	2(6%)
Microwaves	40	21(52.5%)	19(47.5%)	–
Ultrasound	30	13(43%)	15(50%)	2(7%)
Ultratherm	30	8(27%)	20(66%)	2(7%)

* 'Healthy' = no complaints, free movements. 'Different degrees of improvement' = considerable reduction of pain and swelling; movements almost normal

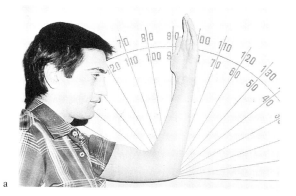
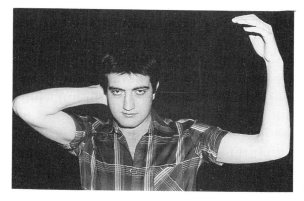

a

b

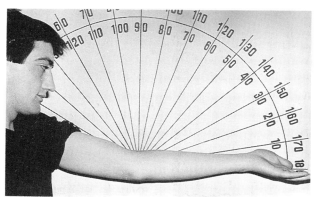
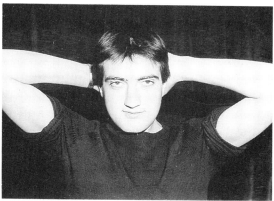

c

d

Fig. 10.55 Patient with loss of range of flexion-extension of the left elbow joint after contusion. a,b. Before IC treatment. c,d. After treatment, showing repair of function.

ultrasound were applied, with restoration of function and dispersion of calcium deposits within 15 days (Fig. 10.56).

Sprains

As a rule treatment of sprains is determined by the severity of the lesion. When joint ligaments are merely stretched, the affected joint is immobilised for 1 to 2 weeks in a light plaster, a splint or a firm bandage. The task of physiotherapy is not difficult in these cases. However, if rupture of the joint ligaments occurs, treatment is more difficult. Preference is always given to conservative treatment (a plaster splint for 1 to 2 months and physiotherapy).

Agreement has not been reached so far as to which of the physiotherapeutic methods gives the best results. Some authors in the past gave preference to diadynamic current, others to

microwaves. Interferential therapy was recommended by a number of authors more than 30 years ago. Steinbach (1961) pointed out its more marked analgesic effect compared with diadynamic current, and Paleirah et al (1956) commented that treatment failed only when the sprain was accompanied by a partial fracture (crack). Thailhades (1959) claimed that IC gave convincing results in sports injuries when 'rapid recovery' was required and the time factor was therefore of primary importance. This is also confirmed by our observations.

Interferential therapy has been applied by us since 1963 using the following methods: 4-plate electrodes of an area of 50 or 100 cm^2 (depending on the size of the affected joint) are placed in such a manner that the two medium-frequency currents cross in the area of the lesion (Figs 3.1, 6.1 and 6.2). When small joints (fingers, wrist joint, etc.) are involved, the treatment is applied with

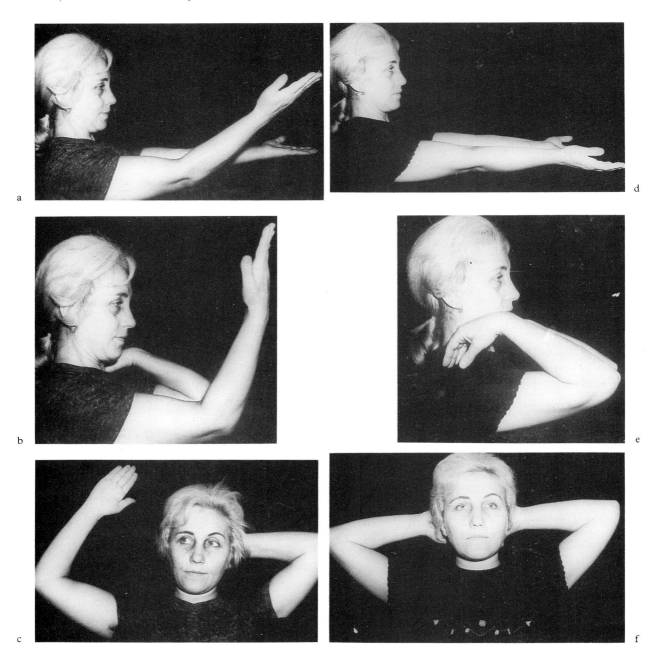

Fig. 10.56 Patient with loss of range of flexion-extension of the right elbow joint after contusion. a,b,c. Before IC and US treatment. d,e,f. After treatment, showing functional restoration.

two 4-field (4-point) electrodes placed transversally across the joint. They can also be positioned longitudinally if there is superficial pain. Interferential current at a rhythmical frequency of 0–100 Hz is applied daily for 15 minutes for a total of 2 to 15 to 20 treatments or more depending on the severity of the case.

A rhythmical frequency of 0–100 Hz is selected because of its analgesic effect, the ability quickly to eliminate toxic metabolic products, to disperse oedema and haematoma and to normalise tissue trophicity.

A total of 235 patients aged between 15 and 66 were given IT, 35 of them receiving IC alternated with microwaves every other day; 158 patients had a lesion of the ankle joint, 30 of the knee joint, 25 of the shoulder, 20 of the elbow and 2 of the wrist. All the patients were admitted with severe pain, oedema and restricted mobility of the affected joint. Treatment started on the 2nd to the 4th day after the injury in 75 patients (treated with rest or a firm bandage), and in the remainder after immobilisation (in 85 patients after 10 to 15 days, and in 75 1 to 3 months after injury).[20] Eighty patients had been given previous treatment with microwaves, diadynamic current and ultratherm.

In 20 patients sprain was combined with marked osteo-arthritis, in 24 with osteoporosis, in 5 with flat foot and in 2 patients there was a free bone fragment. In other words additional complications in 51 patients interfered with recovery. Thirty-four patients suffered from severe sprains.

We have found that, from the first treatments with IC, improvement takes place, pain subsides, oedema decreases and movements increase. In mild cases of sprain complaints can disappear after only 2 to 3 treatments, if treatment is started within the first 24 hours. Patients with complica-

[20] In cases of longer duration and extremely restricted movements, a rhythmical frequency of 0–10 Hz can be alternated with the frequency of 0–100 Hz.

tions such as concomitant osteoporosis and osteo-arthritis require a greater number of treatments (Nikolova, 1966c, 1967b, 1971a). Comparative studies show better results with IT than with any other physiotherapeutic methods (Table 10.12). The particular advantage of IC as compared with microwaves and ultrasound is that it can be applied in osteoporosis and slight fractures (cracks) and that it can disperse pathological calcium deposits.

Long-term results (up to 1 year later) were followed up in 50 patients. No complaints were found. The beneficial effect of IC can be illustrated by the following example:

A 37-year-old patient fell on his left arm. A left elbow joint sprain was diagnosed and the arm was placed in a plaster slab for 7 days. Because of strongly restricted and painful movements (40° in the elbow joint), diadynamic current was prescribed. After 10 ineffective applications, treatment was continued with IC. The patient was relieved of pain after the 10th treatment and complete restoration of function was reached after 20 treatments (Fig. 10.57).

As a rule, in cases of sprain, we do not apply passive movements and massage which, according to a number of authors (Böhler, 1938; Nikolova, 1969a, 1971d; Nikolova & Balchev, 1972), are responsible for the appearance of periarticular ossifications and rigidities, in particular, in the area of the elbow joint. Similar or other complications are absent when interferential therapy is used, and IT also greatly improves metabolism

Table 10.12 Comparison of IT and other methods in treating sprains

Applied therapeutic method	Number of patients	Therapeutic results*		
		Healthy	Different degrees of improvement	No effect
IC	200	150(75%)	50(25%)	–
IC and microwaves	35	29(83%)	6(17%)	–
Microwaves	56	30(53%)	26(47%)	–
Diadynamic current	100	30(30%)	65(65%)	5(5%)
Ultratherm	45	8(18%)	33(73%)	4(9%)
Ultrasound	25	3(12%)	18(72%)	4(16%)

* 'Healthy' = removal of pain and swelling, normal movements. 'Different degrees of improvement' = considerable relief of pain, reduction of swelling, movements almost normal

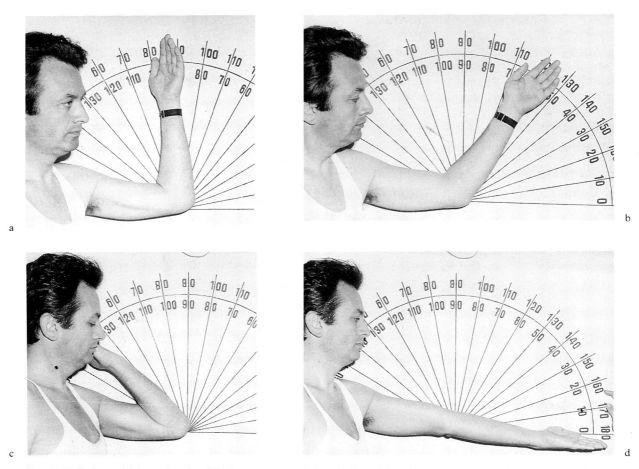

Fig. 10.57 Patient with loss of range of flexion-extension of the left elbow joint after a sprain. a,b. Before treatment with IC. c,d. After treatment, showing restoration of function.

and normalises tissue trophicity, thus helping to prevent the undesirable complications mentioned above. We therefore recommend its early application without waiting for the effect of other physiotherapeutic methods.

Isolated traumatic injury of the tibiofibular syndesmosis

Treatment is conducted in the same manner as in sprain of the ankle joint. We have applied IT for the first time in 20 patients (all with a typical radiograph showing ankle diastasis) after removal of plaster. Interferential current is advisable because of its analgesic effect. By regulating tissue

trophicity, it helps to heal ligaments completely between the tibia and fibula and to normalise the function of the ankle joint (Nikolova & Gerchev, 1972).

Dislocations

The basic treatment for traumatic dislocation of joints is reduction of the displacement, which should be done as soon as possible. Immediately after immobilisation, pain should be relieved, inflammatory signs and haemorrhage eliminated and normal movements restored. A number of physical agents — electrotherapeutic and kinesitherapeutic — are very useful, though the results expected are not always attained. The result depends on how much tissue has been traumatised during reduction and on the correct rehabilitation programme.

No data are available in the literature on the effect of IT in rehabilitation of traumatic dislocations. We have applied it since 1963 independently or in combination with other methods. We have observed 80 patients (46 men and 34 women) within a 6- to 10-year period. The site of the dislocation is presented in Table 10.13. Forty-two patients were admitted with stiffness of the joint and pain immediately after immobilisation. The remaining 38 patients had been given previous treatment with baths, ultrasound and paraffin applications, all of which had failed.

Interferential therapy was applied as for a sprain. As soon as the pain subsided, IC at a rhythmical frequency of 0–10 Hz was used combined with remedial exercises. Complete restoration of function was obtained mainly in patients with early and careful reduction and early application of IC. The very first and immediate effect of IC was reduction or relief of pain (Nikolova, 1970b,e). This allows the early inclusion of remedial exercises, which are essential for a more rapid and complete restoration of function.

The beneficial effect of IC manifests itself most rapidly when applied in lesions of the shoulder and elbow joints, usually after 10 to 15 treatments. The following examples illustrate the excellent results obtained with IC:

A 20-year-old student fell and sustained a dislocation of the right elbow joint which, after reduction, was immobilised in plaster for 15 days. After removal of the plaster, the patient had pain and movements were greatly restricted (Fig. 10.58). She was admitted to our Clinic and given 3 IC treatments at a constant frequency of 100 Hz and 12 treatments with a rhythmical frequency of 0–100 Hz. Complete recovery of function was attained (Fig. 10.58c,d).

Table 10.13 Site of dislocation

Affected joint	Number of patients
Shoulder	20
Elbow	40
Hip	6
Knee	8
Ankle	6

A 22-year-old patient fell on his left arm on October 15th, 1976 and in spite of the severe pain did not immediately see a doctor. As the pain got worse, he consulted a traumatologist the following day. The condition was not diagnosed, however. About 5 months later it was established that he had sustained an acromioclavicular dislocation, which accounted for the subjective complaints. A supporting elastic-compression bandage was made with an Esmarch's bandage and was applied for 56 days. After removal of fixation, limitation of flexion-extension of the elbow joint and abduction-elevation in the shoulder joint were noted as sequelae of long immobilisation (Fig. 10.59a,b,c). Interferential current was applied in combination with US, which ensured complete repair of function (Fig. 10.59d,e,f).

A 16-year-old patient was admitted with a diagnosis of loss of range following dislocation of the right elbow (Fig. 10.60a,b). After 20 treatments with IC complete recovery of function was reached (Fig. 10.60c,d).

A further example illustrates that IT does not always result in complete restoration of function:

A 48-year-old patient fell on September 17th, 1975 and sustained a dislocation of the right shoulder. It was reduced by the orthopaedist-traumatologist. The X-ray taken the same day showed a fracture of the greater tuberosity (Fig. 10.61a). The arm was supported by a sling. The patient was sent to our Clinic for physiotherapy with a diagnosis of dislocated right shoulder, fractured tuberosity and calcification in the right deltoid muscle (Fig. 10.61b). She complained of violent pain and almost completely blocked movements in the shoulder (Fig. 10.62a,b). Satisfactory improvement was reached after 20 treatments with IC (Fig. 10.62c,d). A better result was hardly to be expected because the calcification required surgical removal of the insertional periostitis, which was not contemplated in spite of the follow-up X-ray. The patient was therefore discharged in a satisfactory condition.

Contractures (stiff joints)

Physiotherapeutic methods play an essential part in both prophylaxis and treatment of all types of contractures. Kinesitherapy, hydrotherapy and electrotherapy are applied more or less successfully.

Interferential therapy in treating stiff joints has been used by us since 1963 in the following four ways depending on the local condition:

1. A rhythmical frequency of 0–10 Hz or 0–15 Hz is used in ordinary contractures bearing in mind that it leads to muscle contractions.

2. In patients complaining of severe pain with faulty reduction and delayed callus forma-

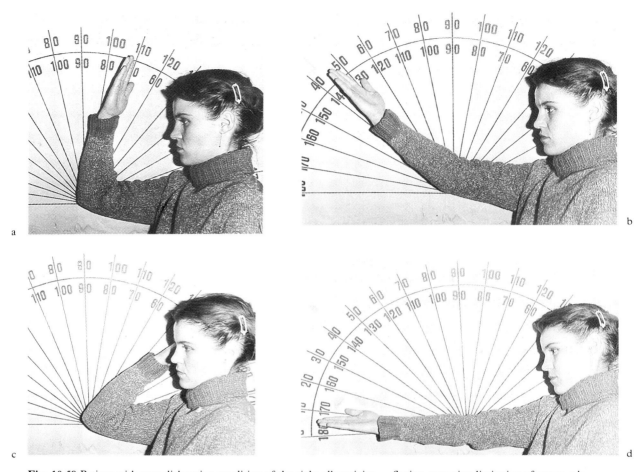

Fig. 10.58 Patient with post dislocation condition of the right elbow joint — flexion-extension limitation of range. a,b. Before treatment with IC. c,d. After treatment, showing restoration of function.

tion, we apply a current at a constant frequency of 100 Hz or a rhythmical frequency of 90–100 Hz (because of their analgesic and antispasmodic effects). Treatment is carried out until pain is relieved and good callus formed.

3. In myositis ossificans, marked haematoma, osteoarthritis and malalignment, a current at a rhythmical frequency of 0–100 Hz is applied because of its analgesic and dispersing effects and the possibility of normalising tissue trophicity.

4. In painful long-standing fractures with malalignment, current at a rhythmical frequency of 0–100 Hz and 0–10 Hz is applied.

Treatment is carried out with 4-plate electrodes (Fig. 6.1b) or 4 vacuum electrodes for 15 minutes. The intensity of the current depends on the patient's tolerance, but he should not experience unpleasant sensations (an overdose has an unpleasant effect). If function is not restored after 15 to 20 treatments, the therapy is resumed after a 5 to 6 day break or is replaced by another physiotherapeutic method, for instance diadynamic current. Interferential therapy leads to restoration of function also when applied independently, but in order to shorten the time of treatment, it should be combined with remedial exercises and other agents, such as ultrasound, after the pain has been relieved, depending on the type of lesion and the joint involved.

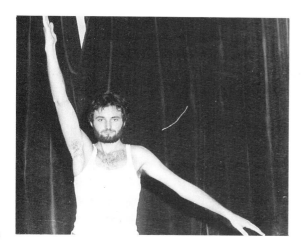

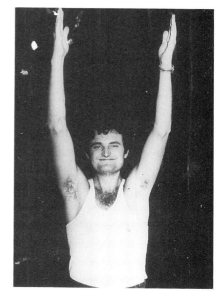

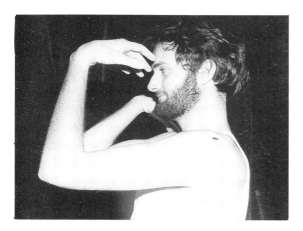

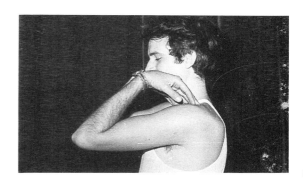

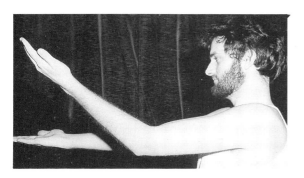

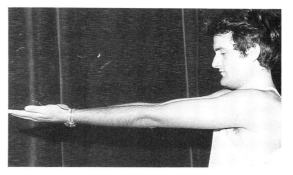

Fig. 10.59 Patient's condition after left acromioclavicular dislocation followed by post immobilisation contractures. a,b,c. Before IC and US treatment. d,e,f. After treatment, showing functional repair.

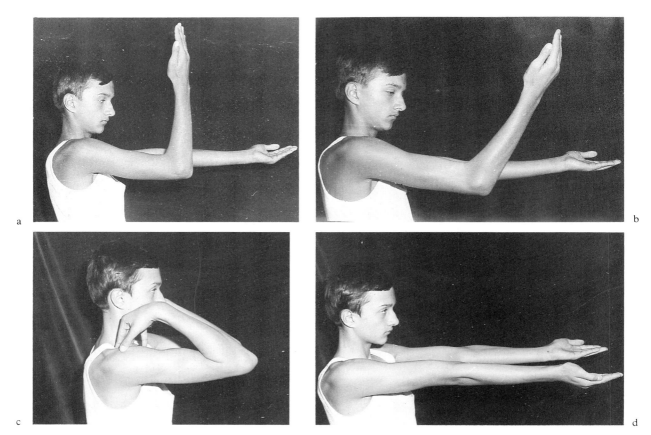

Fig. 10.60 Patient with post dislocation condition of the right elbow joint. a,b. Before IC treatment. c,d. After treatment, showing restoration of function.

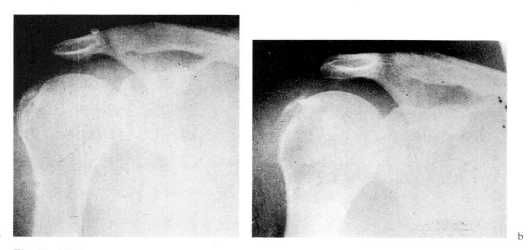

Fig. 10.61 Patient with post dislocation condition of the right shoulder joint. a. X-ray on April 17th, 1975 showed avulsion of the greater tuberosity. b. X-ray check-up on May 14th, 1975 showed calcification in the right deltoid muscle.

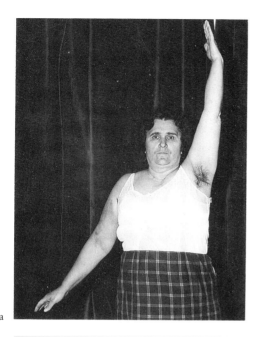

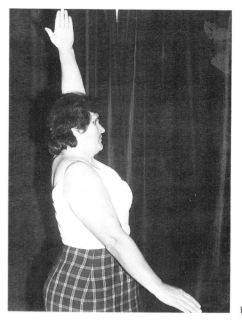

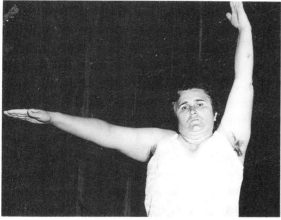

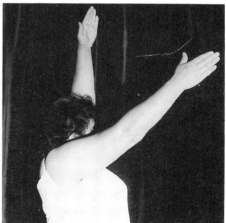

Fig. 10.62 Same patient as in Figure 10.61. a,b. Before treatment with IC. c,d. After treatment, showing satisfactory improvement of function.

For more than 20 years we have observed a great number of post-traumatic stiff shoulders, elbows, hips, knees and ankles. A greater or lesser beneficial effect from using IT was found in all of them. Patients for whom other physiotherapeutic methods had proved unsatisfactory also benefited from IC (Fig. 10.57).

Loss of range of the elbow joint secondary to intra-articular fractures of the head of the radius should be dealt with separately. It can be: (a)

uncomplicated, (b) in combination with other lesions of the elbow joint such as epicondylar fragments and cracks, and (c) in combination with fractures of the humeral diaphysis and some of the forearm bones.

Conservative treatment is recommended at present in undisplaced or slightly displaced fractures of the head of the radius (when the angle of deviation does not exceed 30°). In more severe axial or peripheral dislocations and in comminuted and non-wedged fractures, the method of treatment is more controversial. Some authors recommend active surgical intervention, others are against hasty surgical treatment, claiming that there is a risk of such complications as injury to the radial nerve, cubitus valgus in childhood or myositis ossificans.

In over 50 patients with intra-articular fractures of the head of the radius (5 of them with relative and 11 with absolute indications for operation), IT combined with remedial exercises proved successful even in those patients who had absolute indications for operative intervention (Nikolova, 1971d; Nikolova & Balchev, 1972). In fact IT was much more effective in some fractures with poor alignment of the radial head than in successfully performed operations with good X-ray appearance but loss of pronation and supination. Bearing in mind the risks of operative treatment which have been pointed out by many authors, we think surgery should not be resorted to, even when indicated, before trying IT. Our point of view is supported by the following example:

A 70-year-old patient was admitted with a diagnosis of fracture dislocation of the right head of the radius with non-union and a stiff elbow (Fig. 10.63). The elbow joint was fixed at an angle of 90° after the arm had been placed in plaster for 3 months (the stiff elbow was a result of prolonged immobility). She was offered an operation but refused because of her age. A month of treatment with IC combined with remedial exercises led to restoration of function (Fig. 10.64).

The analysis of this case undoubtedly has shaken the belief in the absolute necessity for surgical treatment in this type of intra-articular lesions and clearly shows the possibilities of rehabilitation with IC in the elderly.

Two further examples illustrate the results of treatment with IT for fracture of the radial head in combination with other lesions:

A 23-year-old patient had an accident on January 5th, 1975 and sustained a fracture. Reduction was attempted the same day but failed. Open reduction with internal fixation was performed two days later and the arm was put in plaster. On March 12th, 1975 the pins were taken out and the arm was immobilised in plaster again. The plaster was removed on April 10th, 1975 and the patient was referred to our Clinic for physiotherapy with a diagnosis of fractured left forearm, fractured left head of radius and left radial epicondyle with a stiff left elbow (Fig. 10.65). The patient had unstable union of the fractures and pain and rigidity of the joints (shoulder, elbow, wrist). Twenty days of IT resulted in complete X-ray and functional recovery (Fig. 10.66d,e,f).

On May 19th, 1976 a 31-year-old patient fell on her left arm, had a violent pain in the whole arm and could not move the elbow joint. Fractures of the ulna and head of the radius were diagnosed. After an unsuccessful attempt at manual reduction, the arm was immobilised in a splint. Because of advanced pregnancy the necessary surgical intervention was postponed until after parturition.

On June 9th, 1976 open reduction of the ulna and metal osteosynthesis were undertaken, followed by plaster

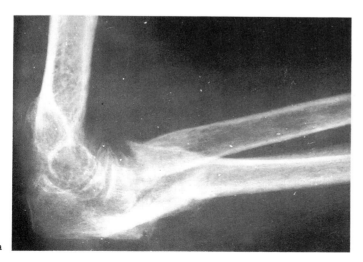
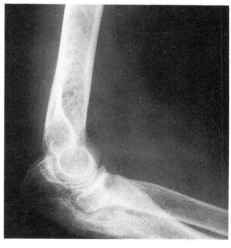

a   b

Fig. 10.63 Patient with fracture-dislocation of the head of the radius. a. X-ray 3 months after the fracture. b. X-ray after 30 days of IT.

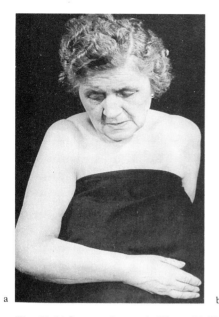 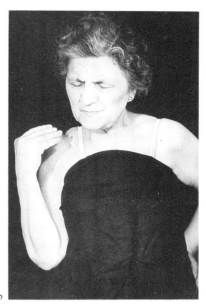 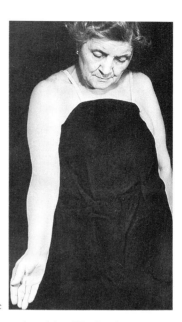

Fig. 10.64 Same patient as in Figure 10.63. Elbow joint fixed at 90°. a. Before IC treatment. b,c. After IT, showing restoration of function.

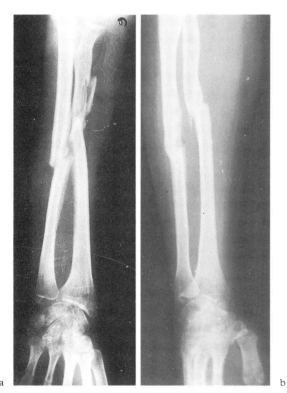

Fig. 10.65 Patient's condition on X-ray after fracture of the forearm and radial head. There is also Sudeck's atrophy of the left hand (see Fig. 10.66).

immobilisation for 2 months. *The plaster was removed on August 4th, 1976.* She was advised that she could do any kind of housework. Her condition deteriorated. A second operation for resection of the head of the radius was performed *on December 27th, 1976* (Fig. 10.67a). The arm was immobilised in a plaster splint for 45 days. Treatment was then carried out with ultrasound, dumb bell lifting and occupational therapy. Ossification appeared in the cubital fossa on each side but not connected with the bones (Fig. 10.67b) resulting from incorrect rehabilitation. Instead of excising the ossification, faulty physiotherapy was continued — baths, massage of the whole arm, passive exercises — which led to further deterioration of her condition with adhesion of the ossification first in the elbow and then in the humerus (Fig. 10.67c) resulting in complete blockage of the joint (total range of movements 10°).

The patient was admitted to our Clinic *on May 30th, 1977,* i.e. a year after the fracture, with flexion-extension contracture of 60°, extension of 50° (Fig. 10.68) and marked hypotrophy of the muscles. Interferential therapy was applied resulting in insignificant improvement of the extension. The flexion did not improve for obvious reasons — the residual bony block of the ulna required surgical removal to release the flexion from the anatomical obstacle.

This case illustrates incorrect physiotherapy prior to operation, and also later when the patient needed further surgical intervention. If the ossification had been removed surgically before bipolar bone adhesions appeared, *the ensuing proper rehabilitation* might have had a better effect, i.e.

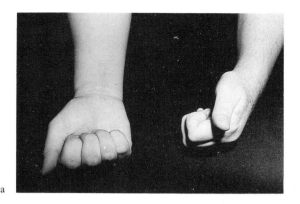

a

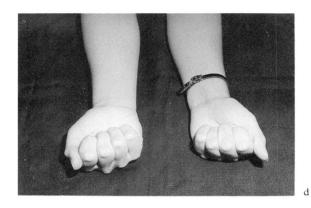

d

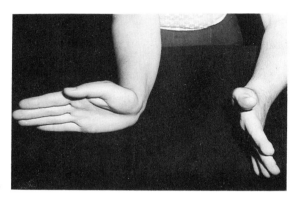

b

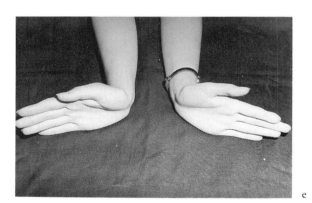

e

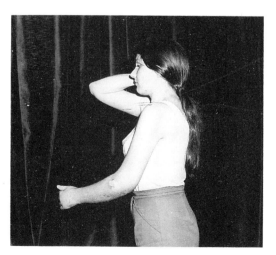

c

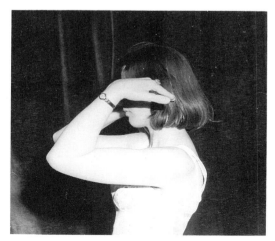

f

Fig. 10.66 Same patient as in Figure 10.65. a,b,c. Before IC treatment — contracture of the elbow joint. d,e,f. After treatment, showing functional repair.

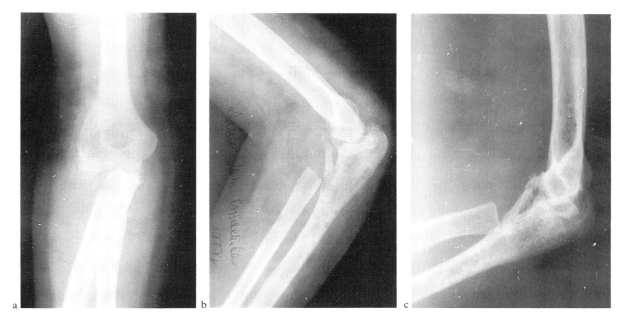

Fig. 10.67 X-rays of the left elbow joint of a patient who had sustained fractures of the ulna and the head of the radius. a. After resection of the head of the radius. b. After treatment with US, lifting dumb-bells and occupational therapy — appearance of ossification in cubital fossa. c. After treatment with baths, massage and passive exercises — union of the ossificate at the humerus and elbow.

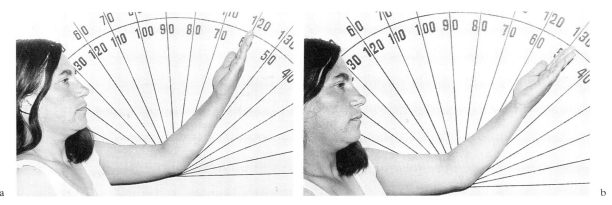

Fig. 10.68 Same patient as in Figure 10.67, showing flexion-extension contracture of the left elbow joint, after wrong physiotherapy. After treatment with IT, flexion still did not improve because of the anatomical obstacle (see text).

dispersion of the residual ossification. It also shows how resection of the radial head might be discredited because of ensuing incorrect rehabilitation.

The effect of IC in traumatic contractures of the elbow joint

Restoration of function in traumatic injuries of the elbow joint is so far an incompletely solved problem. Anatomical and pathophysiological peculiarities of this joint require a more careful rehabilitation, particularly as it has the highest incidence of complications as compared with other joints. Studies on traumatic injuries of elbow joints (Nikolova & Balchev, 1972) suggest that the following causes are responsible for contracture and incomplete recovery of function:

1. Errors of the orthopaedic-traumatologist:

incorrect diagnosis, faulty and incomplete reduction of fractures and dislocations, long-standing cases held in non-physiological extension (olecranon or supracondyle fractures), unsuccessfully selected or technically badly performed surgical procedures. These accounted for 45% of the patients under study.

2. Errors of the physiotherapist: incorrect and ill-founded physiotherapy such as hot baths, mud or paraffin applications, radiant heat, ultratherm, passive movements and massage in the area of the joint, weight-lifting, lack of periodic X-ray check-ups of the effect of treatment, refusal to give physiotherapy because of internal splinting instead of selecting an appropriate treatment. These accounted for 20% of the patients.

3. Combined errors of the orthopaedic-traumatologist and the physiotherapist and lack of effective physiotherapy such as remedial gymnastics and massage of the symmetrical limb and IT, while the patient is in plaster. These accounted for 18% of the patients.

4. Other causes outside the control of the orthopaedic-traumatologist and the physiotherapist: the severity of the trauma itself, cicatricial processes in the capsule and calcification related to the reaction of tissues, myogenic and neurogenic factors. These accounted for 17% of the patients.

It should be stressed that many authors attach more importance to kinesitherapy (active movements, treatment position) in treatment of elbow contractures and *underestimate* other physiotherapeutic methods, especially modern electrotherapeutic methods such as interferential current, ultrasound and diadynamic current, because they are not familiar enough with their therapeutic effects.

Pain greatly interferes with early movements of the elbow joint. It makes the patient spare the joint, muscle spasm is increased and movements are not performed to maximum full range. The electrotherapeutic methods referred to above contribute to relief of pain and muscle spasm, improve the blood circulation and selectively

influence the autonomic nervous system. They are therefore used in a variety of joint contractures, including elbow contracture, but not always in time in spite of the fact that we proved long ago that IT applied independently or in combination with remedial exercises substantially contributes to combating pain and restoring function in all types of traumatic injuries of joints (Nikolova, 1966c, 1971a,d).

Given the absence of unanimity on the effect of electrotherapeutic methods in traumatic contractures of the elbow joint, we set ourselves the task of making a comparative study on the effect of IC, diadynamic current and ultrasound, as well as on the effect of the simultaneous and consecutive application of IC and ultrasound.

Our observations for the period from 1972 to 1979 cover a total of 184 patients with contractures of the elbow joint, aged between 5 and 72 years (74 men, 68 women and 42 children aged between 5 and 14).

Traumatic injury of the elbow joint was caused by: intra-articular fractures (34%), dislocations (17%), contusion or sprain of the elbow joint (12%), supracondylar fractures (11%) and post-traumatic loss of range secondary to prolonged immobilisation of the upper extremity after fractures of the shoulder and the forearm (26%). In 80 of the patients under observation (43%) a number of errors were made in therapy (Table 10.14). As a result, no improvement was obtained in 31 patients, the condition of the loss of range deteriorated in 26 patients and an additional complication — myositis ossificans — developed in 19. Faulty reduction was diagnosed in 35 patients (20%) and concomitant Sudeck's atrophy and delayed callus formation in 15 patients (7 of them with metal implants).

Table 10.14 Physiotherapeutic errors in treating traumatic contractures of the elbow joint

Unsuitable applied therapeutic method	Number of patients
Hot baths, paraffin applications, fomentations	26
Shortwave – thermal dose	14
Thermotherapy plus massage of the joint	10
Thermotherapy and passive gymnastics, weightlifting, hanging on hands	30

The patients were distributed into five groups according to the five methods of treatment under investigation (Table 10.15) and the groups were closely matched with respect to the trauma.

Interferential therapy was applied at a constant frequency of 100 Hz or a rhythmical frequency of 0–100 Hz for 15 minutes daily for a total of 12 to 15 treatments.

Treatment with diadynamic current was provided in such a manner that the electrodes were placed transversally across the joint, first anteroposterioly then from side to side. The short-period modulation was used, the pole being changed in the middle of the procedure. There were 15 treatments in a therapeutic course.

Treatment with US was applied using the labile technique at a frequency of 800 kHz and 0.3–0.5 W/cm^2 for 6 to 12 minutes, for a total of 10 to 12 applications. In 24 patients US was applied to the affected area between the IT electrodes actually during the application of IC. In 40 patients IC and US were applied consecutively, i.e. first IC, then US immediately afterwards (Table 10.15).[21]

[21] As soon as the pain subsided, remedial exercises were applied simultaneously in all patients. They included only careful active movements, without any passive correction. We have studied the independent effect of remedial exercises (Nikolova, 1983) and have found that they do relieve pain and help to eliminate the stiff condition mainly in good reductions, but not as rapidly as IC (Fig. 10.69b).

The results were assessed using the following parameters: subjective complaints of the patients and their progression, goniometry, centimetry, dynamometry and X-ray examination; they were then classifed as 'excellent', 'good', 'satisfactory' and 'poor' (see Table 10.15).

The effect of treatment in the five groups of patients is shown in Table 10.15 and Figure 10.69a. Clearly the best results were obtained by the three groups of patients treated with IC, and IC with ultrasound[22] The effect on one of the basic indices — range of movement — is of great statistical significance ($p < 0.001$). The same is true of dynamometry ($p < 0.001$).

The better functional results obtained with IC, when used alone, or when applied simultaneously or consecutively with US, can be explained by its more marked analgesic effect and its ability rapidly to disperse oedema and haematomata and to normalise metabolic processes. On the other hand, the combination of IC with ultrasound

[22] Satisfactory results in these 3 groups of patients were obtained in intra-articular fractures (11 patients — 7 of them with myositis ossificans); malalignment (8 patients) and concomitant traumatic neuritis (9 patients). Bearing in mind these objective changes, the satisfactory results are also a therapeutic success!
Patients who did not respond to or were only slightly influenced by diadynamic current or US were then given IC followed by US, which led to removal of the contracture and to essential improvement in the useful function of the joint in cases of malalignment and other complications.

Table 10.15 Comparison of IT and other methods in treating traumatic contractures of the elbow joint

Applied therapeutic method	Number of patients	Therapeutic results*			
		Excellent	Good	Satisfactory	Poor
IC (Group I)	76	32(42%)	27(36%)	17(22%)	–
Diadynamic current (Group II)	24	4(17%)	7(29%)	9(37%)	4(17%)
US (Group III)	20	3(15%)	5(25%)	7(35%)	5(25%)
Simultaneous IC and US (Group IV)	24	13(54%)	6(25%)	4(17%)	1(4%)
Consecutive IC and US (Group V)	40	22(55%)	10(25%)	7(17.5%)	1(2.5%)

* 'Excellent' = patients with complete restoration of function. 'Good' = patients without subjective complaints and insignificant loss in the range of movement, i.e. extension to 10–15° at complete supination and pronation. 'Satisfactory' = patients with still persisting subjective complaints, flexion contracture to 40°, limitation of pronation and supinatin movements. 'Poor' = patients who had neither subjective nor objective changes in their condition after treatment

undoubtedly results in mutual enhancement of their therapeutic effects (Nikolova, 1979).

At present the consecutive application of IC and ultrasound is to be recommended. In fact, it is very similar in effect to their simultaneous application as US follows immediately after IC and affects tissues already influenced by IC.

The following are some examples to illustrate the results obtained:

> On January 23rd, 1977 this patient fell and sustained a fracture of the right humerus at the shoulder. The arm was placed in plaster for 5 months. She was then treated with mud applications, remedial exercises, massage and occupational therapy. However, her condition did not improve, so she was referred to our Clinic on August 8th, 1977 (more than 6 months after the fracture). The diagnosis was loss of range of movement of the elbow joint and rigidity of the shoulder joint (Fig. 10.70a,b) Interferential therapy and ultrasound were used in sequence, resulting in restoration of function (Fig. 10.70c,d).

A 7-year-old patient was admitted with a diagnosis of left supracondylar fracture of the humerus and loss of elbow range 4 months after a fracture (Fig. 10.71a.b.c).

Treatment with IT led to restoration of joint function (Fig.10.71d,e).

On November 30th, 1973 a 50-year-old patient was examined by an orthopaedic-traumatologist because of contusion of the left elbow joint. No fracture was detected in the X-ray. A second X-ray examination was made on December 17th, 1973 because of persisting pain and swelling in the area of the joint, and this revealed a fracture of the left head of the radius with a stiff elbow joint (Fig. 10.72a). She was referred for interferential therapy and a total of 12 treatments were carried out. The control X-ray did not detect any changes except for a slight deformity of the radial head. Function was restored (Fig. 10.72b).

A 22-year-old patient had an accident on October 1st, 1977. The arm was put in a plaster after reduction the same day, and the plaster was removed on October 22nd, 1977. The patient was referred to our Clinic on October 31st, 1977 with a diagnosis of dislocation of the left elbow and fractured head of the radius and stiff left elbow (Fig. 10.73a-c) with a bone fragment from the medial condyle of the left humerus. Interferential therapy was applied followed by US, for a total of 16 treatments. Function was restored, the extension being only slightly restricted.

A 15-year-old patient sustained a fracture on January 2nd, 1979 and the affected arm was immobilised in plaster

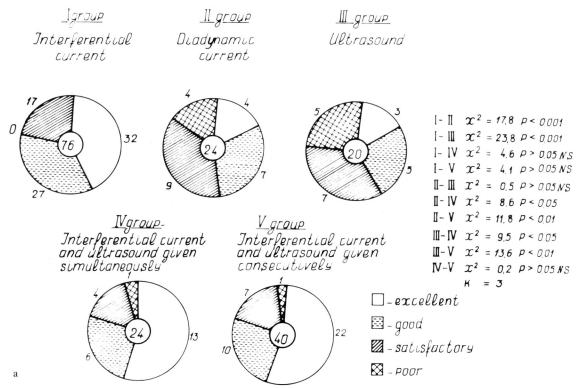

a

Fig. 10.69 Comparative therapeutic results in treating elbow contracture. a. Various methods compared.

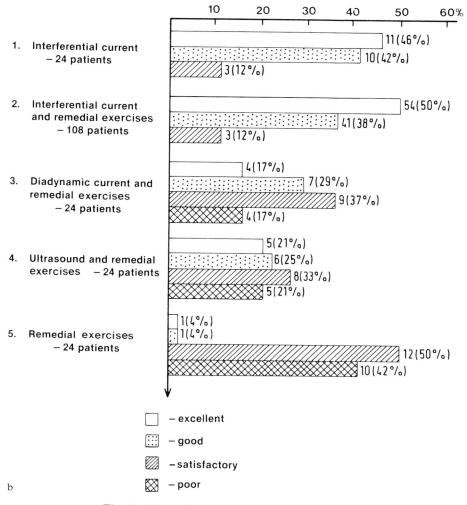

1. Interferential current
   – 24 patients

   11 (46%)
   10 (42%)
   3 (12%)

2. Interferential current
   and remedial exercises
   – 108 patients

   54 (50%)
   41 (38%)
   3 (12%)

3. Diadynamic current and
   remedial exercises
   – 24 patients

   4 (17%)
   7 (29%)
   9 (37%)
   4 (17%)

4. Ultrasound and remedial
   exercises   – 24 patients

   5 (21%)
   6 (25%)
   8 (33%)
   5 (21%)

5. Remedial exercises
   – 24 patients

   1 (4%)
   1 (4%)
   12 (50%)
   10 (42%)

☐ – excellent

▦ – good

▨ – satisfactory

▩ – poor

b

Fig. 10.69 (contd.) b. The effect of remedial exercises.

for 57 days. She was admitted for rehabilitation on March 5th, 1979 with a diagnosis of left Colles' fracture and stiff elbow (Fig. 10.74a,b,c) Interferential therapy was carried out followed consecutively by US, resulting in restoration of function (Fig. 10.74d,e,f).

A 12-year-old patient sustained a fracture of the arm on February 28th, 1979 which was immobilised in plaster. She was referred to our Clinic for rehabilitation on April 4th, 1979 with a diagnosis of fractured neck of the right radius and stiff right elbow (Fig. 10.75a,b). Interferential therapy was applied alternating with ultrasound for 17 days and resulted in restoration of function (Fig. 10.75c,d).

Our observations make it possible to draw the following conclusions, which are very important for clinical practice:

1. Interferential current is the most effective treatment of contractures of the elbow joint following fractures and other injuries of soft tissues as compared with diadynamic current and US. In our study complete restoration of function was obtained in 42% of patients against 17% for diadynamic current and 15% for ultrasound (Table 10.15). Better results were also obtained when IC was applied in treating contracture of the elbow joint with concomitant myositis ossificans.

2. In our study satisfactory results were obtained in the treatment of elbow contrac-

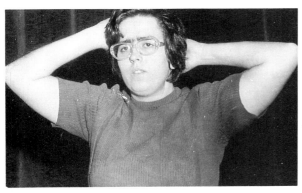
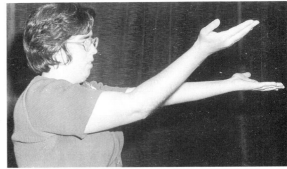

a

b

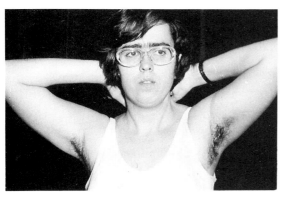
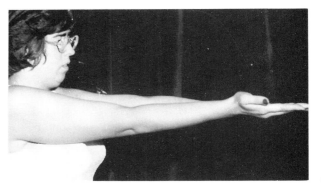

c

d

Fig. 10.70 Patient with flexion-extension contracture of the elbow joint after fracture of the right humerus. a,b. Before IC and US treatment given consecutively. c,d. After treatment, showing functional repair.

tures for 22% of patients treated with IC, for 37% treated with diadynamic current and 35% treated with ultrasound (Table 10.15). Most of these patients had complicated traumatic injuries of the bony framework of the elbow and of the soft tissues (incomplete reduction, injury of peripheral nerves, myositis ossificans).

3. Another advantage of IC is that it can be applied safely with metal implants.

4. The best results are obtained in all methods when treatment starts immediately after immobilisation or not later than the third week.

5. The results are most convincing when IC and ultrasound are applied consecutively. In our study there was complete restoration of function in 55% of patients (Table 10.15).

Tuberculosis of bones and joints

No data are available in the literature on the application of IC in the treatment of tuberculosis of bones and joints. We apply IC at a rhythmical frequency of 0–100 Hz after arthroplasty, for a total of 15 to 25 treatments for 15 minutes daily. It contributes to relief of pain and improves the condition of the musculoskeletal mechanism.

Flat foot

By chance we noticed the positive effect of IC in static flat foot while treating patients with Sudeck's atrophy and osteoarthritis of the ankle joint combined with flat foot. The effect is due to the analgesic action of interferential current with resultant improvement in tissue trophicity and strengthening of muscles. Treatment is applied

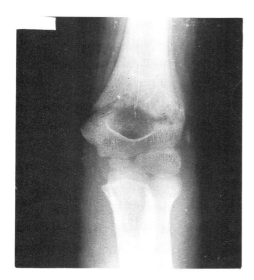

a

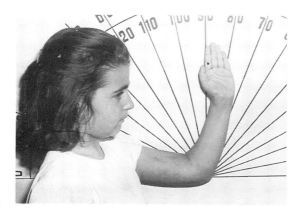

b

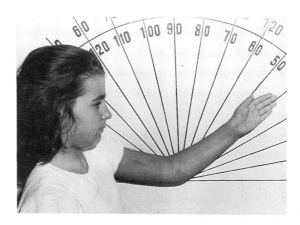

c

Fig. 10.71 Patient's condition after supracondylar fracture of the humerus. a,b,c. Before therapy with IC; the X-ray (a) shows a clear fracture line. d,e. After treatment, showing repair of function.

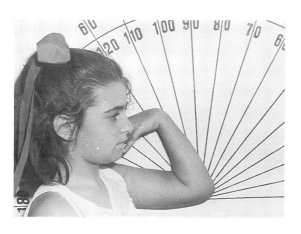

d

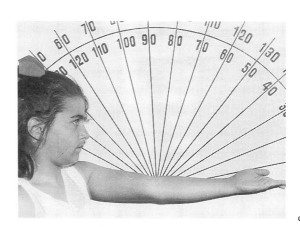

e

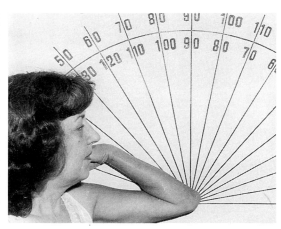

a   b

Fig. 10.72 Patient with contracture of the left elbow after fracture of the radial head. a. Before treatment with IC. b. After treatment, showing restoration of function.

with 4-plate electrodes placed in such a manner that the foot is in the interference area of the two component currents. A constant frequency of 100 Hz is applied in the first 3 treatments, followed by a rhythmical frequency of 0–100 Hz for 15 minutes daily, for a total of 20 to 25 treatments. Especially good results are obtained if the interference vector is applied in combination with vacuum massage. In general, interferential therapy can be successfully combined with other physiotherapeutic methods (e.g. microwaves, alternated every other day) and of course with padding of the arches.

Intra-articular fractures

Interferential therapy in the treatment of closed intra-articular fractures is started immediately after reduction to relieve pain and to stimulate callus formation. It is applied at a constant frequency of 90–100 Hz for 15 minutes daily, for a total of 20 treatments. When treatment is started later, e.g. after removal of immobilisation (in closed and open intra-articular fractures), and fibrous adhesions are present in joints and soft tissues, the rhythmical frequency is selected at 0–100 Hz. The chances of a better recovery are considerably improved.

Interferential current is successfully applied in treating loose bodies in the joint in the post-operative period. A constant frequency is applied in the first 2 to 5 treatments, and a frequency of 0–100 Hz in the remainder for 15 to 20 minutes, for a total of 10 to 20 treatments.

Hallux valgus

We have applied interferential current in 20 patients with hallux valgus (6 patients in the initial stage, and 14 postoperatively). In patients in the initial stage pain relief was obtained on average after 6 to 10 treatments. Rapid pain relief and restoration of function were also achieved in the surgical patients.

Interferential current is applied with 4 small-plate electrodes at a constant frequency of 100 Hz in the first 3 treatments, followed by a rhythmical frequency of 0–100 Hz; if a concomitant osteoporosis is present, however, only a constant frequency is selected.

Lesions of the ligaments of the knee

Interferential current in the treatment of partially lacerated or merely stretched lateral and cruciate ligaments of the knee is applied during the immobilisation period, at a rhythmical frequency of 0–100 Hz. It helps to disperse haematomata, relieve pain and improve tissue trophicity. The electrodes are placed as in knee joint arthritis

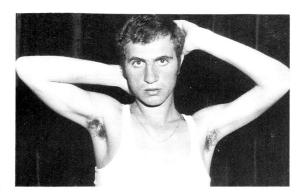

a

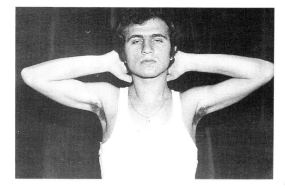

d

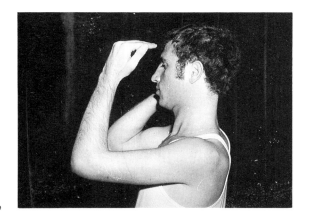

b

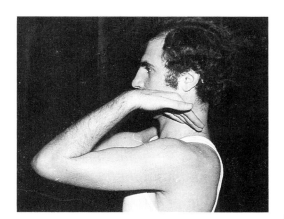

e

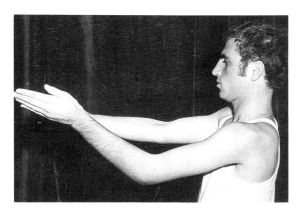

c

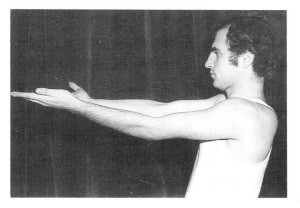

f

Fig. 10.73 Patient with post-traumatic contracture of the left elbow joint. a,b,c. Before IC and US given consecutively. d,e,f. After treatment, showing nearly perfect restoration of function

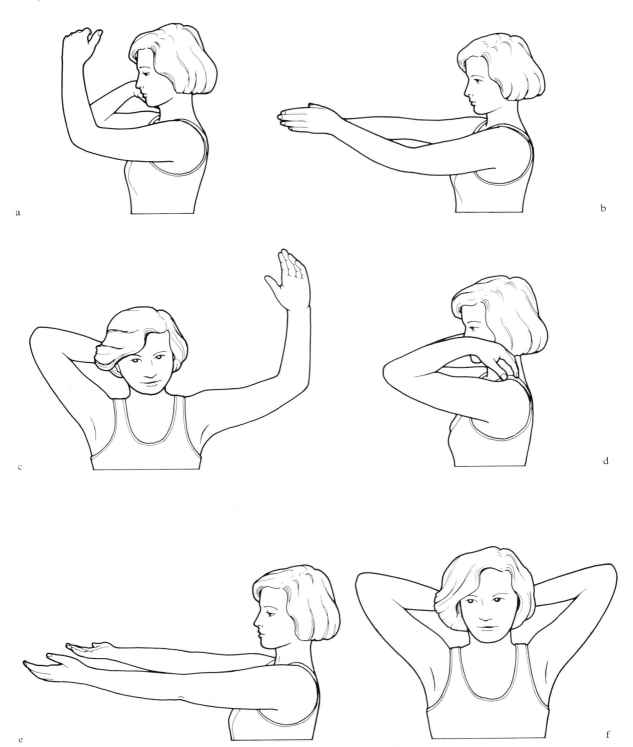

Fig. 10.74 Contracture of the left elbow joint after Colles' fracture. a,b,c. Before IC and US given consecutively. d,e,f. After treatment, showing restoration of function.

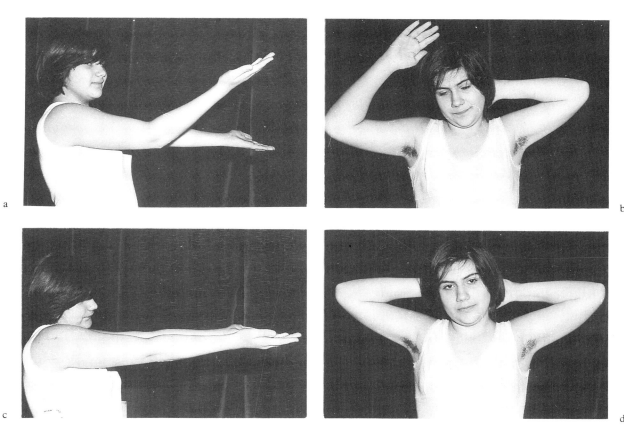

Fig. 10.75 Patient with contracture of the right elbow joint. a,b. Before IC and US given consecutively. c,d. After treatment, showing restoration of function.

(Figs 3.1 and 6.3), and treatments are carried out daily for 15 to 20 minutes, with a total of 15 in a therapeutic course.

Timely surgical treatment is required in complete laceration of the ligaments. IC is then applied in the same manner as in partially lacerated ligaments. Very good results are obtained when IC is combined with vacuum or vibration massage and appropriate remedial exercises.

Injuries of the menisci

Timely surgical treatment, i.e. removal of the injured meniscus, is considered to be the only radical method of treatment. Complete restoration of function, however, is brought about not only by a timely and well-performed operation but also by postoperative rehabilitation. Remedial

exercises and massage are of primary importance in this respect. Electrophoresis with Novocain and KI, shortwave, etc., are also recommended.

Postoperative IT was introduced by us as early as 1964. A total of 80 patients (43 men and 37 women, 44 patients aged between 16 and 30, 32 between 31 and 50, and 4 above 50) were under observation. The period of time from the injury to the operation was as follows: 1 to 2 months — 27 patients; 3 to 6 months — 29 patients; 6 to 8 months — 9 patients; 9 to 12 months — 9 patients; and over 1 year — 6 patients. The medial meniscus was injured in 53 patients, the lateral in 22 and both the medial and the lateral in 5 patients. Concomitant osteo-arthritis of the knee joint was found in 8 patients, a foreign body in 5 patients, laceration of the anterior cruciate ligament in 4, chondromalacia in 5 patients, and calcium deposits in 3 patients. Forty patients had sports injuries, 39 patients home and traffic accidents and 1 patient a gunshot injury. The commencement of treatment is indicated in Table 10.16.

Previous treatment, including paraffin applications, massage, baths and microwave, was used in 15 of the patients. We applied IC and remedial exercises in 40 patients, and IC with microwave or ozocerite applications in the rest of the patients. A constant frequency of 100 Hz was applied during the first 2 to 3 treatments followed by a rhythmical frequency of 0–100 Hz. In cases of severe pain a constant frequency of 100 Hz and a rhythmical frequency can be provided for 10 minutes daily. In concomitant Sudeck's atrophy only a constant frequency of 100 Hz is applied. Specially good (excellent) results are obtained when IC is alternated with ultrasound.

The immediate result of IC is relief of pain and improved movements (Nikolova, 1970c, 1979). Complete restoration of functions usually occurs after a total of 20 treatments. The clinical analysis enabled us to draw the following conclusions:

1. Interferential current administered to patients following a meniscectomy results in rapid relief of pain and elimination of inflammation and haematomata; it also allows more favourable conditions for remedial exercises, which are generally recognised as bringing about a more rapid recovery of function.

2. The combination of IC with microwave is especially suitable for the treatment of inflammatory signs, and with ozocerite applications in marked rigidity of joints.

3. In general, the results are better when patients are admitted earlier for operation and when IT is started soon after the operation.

Table 10.16 Time span between operation and commencement of physiotherapeutic treatment for injuries of the menisci

Commencement of treatment	Number of patients
From 10th to 20th postoperative day	48
From 30th to 40th postoperative day	23
Over 4 months to 1 year	9

At present surgical treatment is recommended in *ossification of the menisci*. We have used IC (a rhythmical frequency of 0–100 Hz) in 3 patients with good clinical results (pain relief and restoration of movements), but with no change in the X-ray findings. Treatment was conducted as in osteo-arthritis of the knee joint.

Chondromalacia

Chondromalacia develops as a result of a single or chronic trauma in the knee area involving the cartilaginous surfaces of the knee joint. In mild cases treatment is medical and in severe ones surgical. Paraffin or mud applications and other treatments have been applied so far in combination with graded movements of the knee joint.

We first applied IC and microwaves and decided to test their effectiveness by applying the two methods independently or consecutively.

Interferential current was applied at a constant frequency of 100 Hz for 15 minutes daily, for a total of 15 to 20 treatments (Fig. 3.1). Microwave therapy was applied through a sand bag at a dosage of 20–30 W for 8 to 15 minutes daily, with 15 treatments altogether.

A total of 160 patients (62 men and 98 women) have been observed since 1966. The patients were aged as follows: 17 patients between 10 and 20 years; 76 between 21 and 40; 63 between 41 and 60; 4 over 60 years. Acute sports trauma and home accidents were established in 134 patients and chronic trauma in 26. Previous medication and other treatment had been provided in the case of 105 patients and operative treatment in 14. The therapeutic results are presented in Table 10.17. They show the greater effectiveness of IC when combined with microwaves and administered every other day.

The beneficial therapeutic effect can be accounted for by the pronounced vasodilating action of IC and microwaves, relieving pain and improving tissue trophicity, which is required in this type of closed injury of the knee joint. One should note that in 24 patients pain and oedema were eliminated and movements were completely restored only after the consecutive application of the 3 methods. Patients treated with IC only were followed up for a 6-month period. Recurrence of

Table 10.17 Results of IT and other methods in treating chondromalacia

Applied therapeutic method	Number of patients	Therapeutic results*		
		Healthy	Different degrees of improvement	No effect
IC	70	17(24%)	51(73%)	2(3%)
IC and microwaves	20	7(35%)	13(65%)	–
Microwaves	70	17(24%)	49(70%)	4(6%)

* 'Healthy' = removal of pain and swelling, restoration of the normal extent of movements. 'Different degrees of improvement' = different degrees of reduction of pain, swelling and other clinical symptoms

complaints was found in 15 (21%). Repeated IT also proved very useful.

SOFT TISSUE INJURIES

Closed traumatic injuries (contusion and haematomata)

Interferential current finds an especially successful application in contusions and haematomata. When applied in time, IC helps to prevent some serious complications such as suppuration and myositis ossificans and accelerates complete recovery of function. A total of 50 patients with haematoma were treated (2 of them with massive haematoma of the whole lower leg, 1 in the hip area). Complete restoration of function was achieved after 6 to 15 treatments. The therapy was carried out at a rhythmical frequency of 0–100 Hz with 4-plate electrodes placed so that the haematoma area was at the crossing point of the two medium-frequency currents. Treatments were given daily for 15 to 20 minutes with a total of 10 to 25 treatments depending on the size of the haematoma. The following example illustrates the beneficial effect of the current:

A 27-year-old patient sustained a sprain of the left elbow joint with a massive haematoma. He had used daily fomentations but his condition deteriorated: pain increased and movements in the joint were restricted (Fig. 10.76a). Ten IC treatments led to dispersion of the haematoma and recovery of movements in the elbow joint (Fig. 10.76b).

Two other examples also confirm the beneficial effect of IC:

A 14-year-old patient had an accident on November 14th, 1966 and sustained a fracture. The arm was placed in plaster for 24 days. She was referred to our Clinic, as her

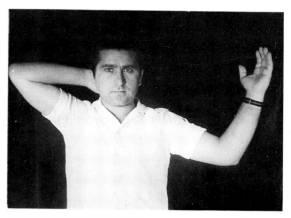

a

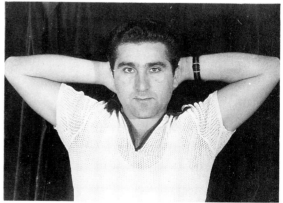

b

Fig. 10.76 Patient with post distortion condition of the left elbow joint with a massive haematoma. a. Before treatment with IC. b. After treatment, showing dispersion of haematoma and repair of function.

condition deteriorated after treatment with baths and massage. The diagnosis was fractured left head of the radius and fracture dislocation of the medial epicondyle with avulsion of the olecranon process and stiff elbow (Fig. 10.77a,b). The volar surface of the cubital fossa was indurated because of a haematoma.

Interferential current was applied at a rhythmical

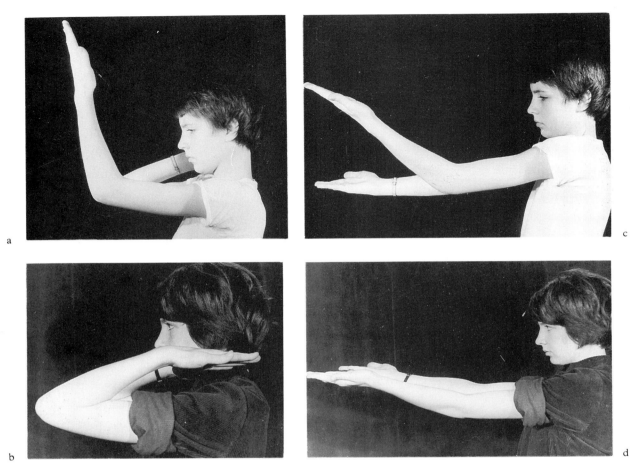

Fig. 10.77 Patient's condition after fracture and haematoma in the area of the left elbow joint. a,b. Before treatment with IC. c,d. After treatment, showing functional restoration.

frequency of 0–100 Hz and 0–10 Hz every other day for a total of 30 treatments. Function was restored (Fig. 10.77c,d) and the haematoma was completely dispersed after the 15th day.

A 20-year-old sportsman fell on April 17th, 1974 and sustained a dislocation of the right elbow joint. An X-ray taken after reduction showed an earlier injury in the same joint with a bone fragment attached to the ulnar epicondyle of the humerus (Fig. 10.78a). He was admitted to our Clinic after immobilisation on May 30th, 1974 with extensive oedema, a haematoma in the cubital fossa and restricted movements of the joint (Fig. 10.78b,c). After 10 treatments with IC the haematoma was dispersed, and after the 20th treatment function of the joint was restored (Fig. 10.78d,e).

Very good results are attained in treating massive hard haematomata when IC is alternated with US, as the following example shows:

A 56-year-old pensioner had been on regular haemodialysis (twice a week) since July 1983 because of bilateral renal polycystosis — chronic renal insufficiency.

During haemodialysis on October 25th, 1983 the needle perforated the cubital artery, which resulted in the formation of a large haematoma on the volar part of the hand. The patient was immediately admitted to hospital for 2 days of treatment — cryotherapy was provided followed by aethacridinum compresses. He was referred to our Clinic for physiotherapy on November 16th, 1983. On examination, a hard haematoma was found involving the left armpit and the area of the elbow fossa. Flexion and extension of the elbow joint and movements of the shoulder joint were restricted. The patient complained of pain in the whole arm. Interferential current followed by ultrasound led to resorption of the haematoma and almost complete restoration of arm function (Fig. 10.79).

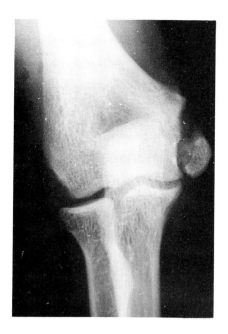

a

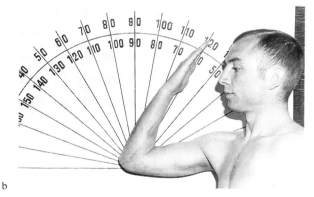

b

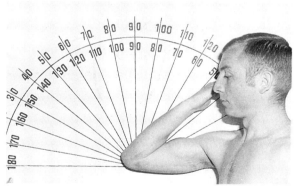

d

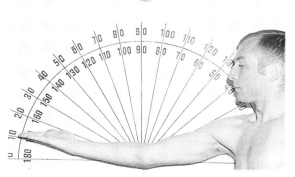

c

e

Fig. 10.78 Patient's condition after right elbow joint dislocation and haematoma in the cubital fossa. a. X-ray of the joint before IC. b,c. Functional ability before treatment with IC. d,e. After treatment, showing repair of function.

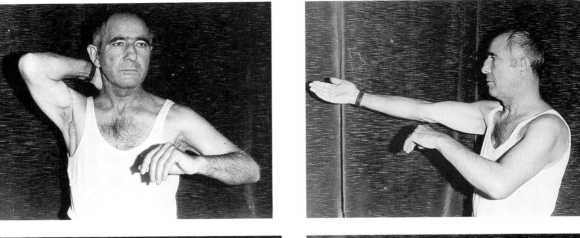

a   b

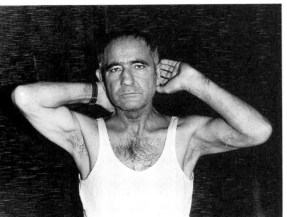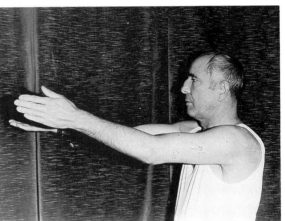

c   d

Fig. 10.79 Contracture of the left elbow joint and rigidity of the shoulder joint after formation of a massive haematoma on the volar side of the hand. a,b. Before IC and US treatment. c,d. After treatment, showing almost complete restoration of function.

Open traumatic injuries (wounds)

Interferential current gives very good results in the treatment of uninfected wounds. Blood circulation improves and epithelisation accelerates, both when IC is applied independently or when IC is applied after the wound has been smeared with a suitable ointment. This beneficial effect was established clinically and also by morphometric and cytomorphological methods in experimentally induced wounds in rats (Nikolova et al, 1984a) as demonstrated by comparing Figures 10.80–10.83 (control groups of rats) with Figures 10.84–10.87 (wounds treated with interferential current).

Interferential therapy is applied with 4-plate electrodes positioned on the intact skin in such a manner that the two currents cross at a point in the wound area. When possible, treatment can also be provided with 2-field electrodes. A current is applied at a rhythmical frequency of 90–100 Hz and 0–100 Hz over a period of 10 to 20 minutes daily, for a total of 15 to 20 treatments. Action upon the segmental area is also recommended at a constant frequency of 100 Hz for 15 minutes daily. An important advantage of the technique is that the electrodes are not in contact with the wounded surface during treatment.

In plantar perforating ulcers, treatment is given to the basic disease, e.g. traumatic injury of the

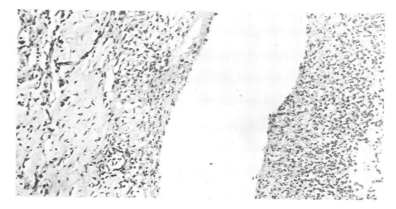

Fig. 10.80 The wound surface is thoroughly covered with massive leukocytic necrotic torus excreting from the underlying tissue. (Stained by haematoxylin-eosin, × 100.)

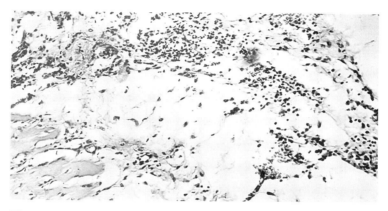

Fig. 10.81 Predominant on the bottom of the wound are the blood cell elements (leukocytes, polynuclears) located among vast necrotic areas. (Stained with H.E., × 75.)

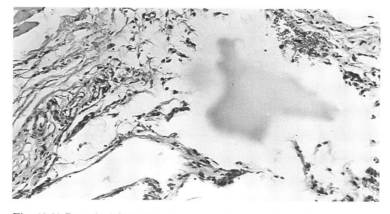

Fig. 10.82 Deposited fibrinoid substances and plasmophagia phenomena are often encountered in necrotic areas. (Stained with H.E., × 75.)

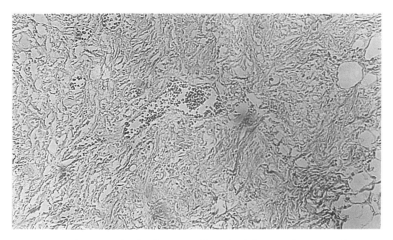

Fig. 10.83 The network of collagenous fibres is delicate and composed mainly of saturn-red positive threads. (Stained after Holosha, × 75.)

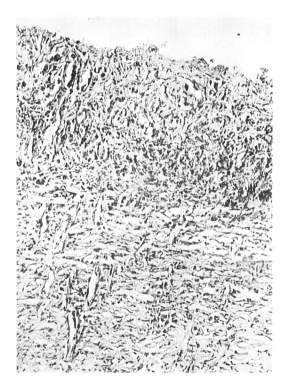

Fig. 10.84 A well-developed epithelial regenerate is seen on the wound surface in the differentiation stage. (Stained with H.E., × 75.)

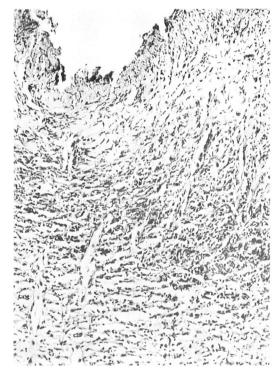

Fig. 10.85 Formation of epidermal layers, including superficial deposition of keratin, is observed in certain areas. (Stained with H.E., × 75.)

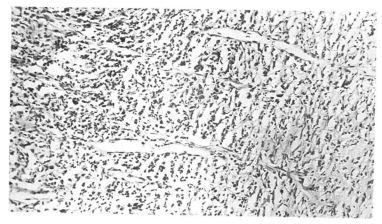

Fig. 10.86 The bottom of the wound is filled by richly vascularised granulation tissue (Stained with H.E., × 75.)

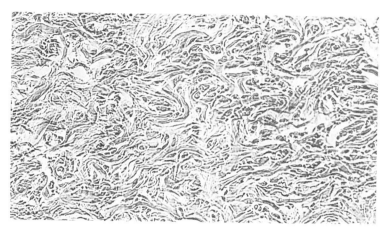

Fig. 10.87 The collagenous network is composed mainly of mature, fuchsin-positive collagenous fibres. (Stained after van Gieson, × 75.)

peripheral nerve or spinal cord disease. Interferential therapy is effective when the whole extremity is treated (Fig. 1.4). The current applied is of a constant frequency of 100 Hz to improve blood circulation, and of a rhythmical frequency of 0–100 Hz to lead to improved tissue trophicity, stimulate nerve regeneration and help epithelisation. A total of 20 treatments are given daily for 15 to 20 minutes. Treatment acting upon the segmental area at a constant frequency of 100 Hz is recommended during a break between 2 therapeutic courses.

Glossary

The following terms occur in the text and may not be familiar to all readers:

Classical methods of diagnosis: old Faradic, Galvanic test, widely used (in English-speaking countries) up to the Second World War, then superseded by a more complete test of the excitability of nerve and muscle, the 'Intensity Duration' or 'Intensity Time Curve'. For further information, readers are referred to *Electrodiagnosis and Electromyography*, 3rd edition, 1971, edited by S. Licht, in particular Chapter 8.

Diadynamic current: various low-frequency currents which are unidirectional, originally used by Bernard, for sensory and motor effects, in the middle of this century.

Electrokinesia: electrical stimulation of muscles.

Electrophoresis: driving medical ions (e.g. KI [potassium iodide], $CaCl_2$, Lydase [Hyaluronidase]) into the skin using a direct current, or iontophoresis.

Head's zones: definite skin areas where reflex pains and hyperalgesia appear in diseases of the internal organs. These skin areas receive their sensitive nerve fibres from the same spinal brain segment as the affected internal organ (e.g. in peptic ulcer, VIII-IX dorsal segment to the left; in biliary colic, VI-IX dorsal segment to the right).

Kymographic insufflation: carbon dioxide is blown through the uterus into the Fallopian tubes for roentgenographic recording of the movements of the organ (Rubin test).

Pallaesthesia: the testing of perception of vibration.

Phonophoresis: driving medical ions (e.g. cortisone) into the skin using ultrasound.

Radon: a colouress, gaseous, radioactive element (obtained by breaking up radium).

Rheography: use of an alternating current of high frequency in order to determine the resistance to blood flow in some particular tissue, e.g. in brain tissue. Method for determining the blood flow in a particular part of the body, e.g. hand, wrist, finger.

Syncardial massage: first introduced in 1945 by M. Fuchs, it is applied through a special apparatus called a 'Syncardon'. Rhythmical pressure impulses by means of a cuff (band) are induced on specific sections of the limbs in order to support and improve the peripheral blood circulation. A novel development in syncardial massage is the inducement of pressure impulses synchronised with the vessel systole of the patient. The duration of the impulses does not exceed the duration of the vessel systole. While these impulses are acting on the vessels, the blood flow in the arteries is increased centrifugally, and in the veins and lymph vessels it is increased centripetally.

References

Arnold W 1978 Bemerkungen für Physiotherapie nach Verletzungen im Ellenbogenbereich. Beiträge zur Orthopädie und Traumatologie 25 (3): 146

Balaba T J, Gurjev W N, Shigalowa L F 1974 Die Bedeutung der Energie-austauschstörungen in der Pathogenese der Arthrosis deformans. Beiträge zur Orthopädie und Traumatologie 21 (3): 128–133

Bernard P et al 1955 Un adjuvant très efficace dans le traitement des contractures post-hémiplégiques. Journal de Radiologie et d'Electrologie 10

de Bisschop G 1958 Über die Stellung der gekreuzten Ströme in der physikalischen Medizin. Elektromedizin 3 (2/3): 1–8

de Bisschop G 1962 A propos de huit ans d'expérience sur les courants de moyenne fréquence. Journal de Radiologie et d'Electrologie 45 (2): 120–122

Böhler L V 1938 Technik der Knochenbruchbehandlung. Maudrich Verlag, Wien

Bozhinov S et al 1973 Myopathies. Medicina i fizkultura Publishing House, Sofia 13–18 (Bulgarian)

Burghart W 1951 Behandlung mit dem Nemectron. Wiener Medizinische Wochenschrift 101 (51–53): 999

Burghart W 1952 Behandlung der Gallenleiden mit dem Nemectron. Wiener Medizinische Wochenschrift 102 (31): 603

Chappelart P 1956 Un traitement physiothérapeutique des migraines. Concours médical 32: 11

Dimitrowa S 1977 Influence of interferential current on oxygen utilization by tissue of patients with obliterating diseases of the peripheral arteries. Voprossi kurortologii, fisioterapii i lechebnoi fisicheskoi kulturi 1: 55–57 (Russian)

de Domenico G 1981 Basic guidelines for interferential therapy. Theramedbooks, Sydney

de Domenico G 1982 Pain relief with interferential therapy. The Australian Journal of Physiotherapy 28 (3): 14–18

Egorov P I, Bogin U N 1961 Application of a new physiotherapeutic method — interference-pulse treatment in internal diseases. Therapevticheskii arkhiv 32 (6): 28–31 (Russian)

Eigler E 1980 Success achieved by treatment with interferential current on patients with epicondylitis humeri. Zeitschrift für physikalische Medizin 9: 7–10

Emminger E 1964 Pathologie der Arthrosis deformans. Physikalische diätetische Therapie 5: 155

Erb W 1882 Handbuch der Elektrotherapie. Leipzig

Fiedler H 1960 Die Interferenzstrombehandlung in Klinik und Praxis. Elektromedizin 5 (1): 1–19

Fournier M, de Bisschop G 1959 Les courants interférés dans le traitement des séquelles de la poliomyélite. Journal de Radiologie et d'Electrologie 40 (10): 586–590

Galin J 1959 Contribution d'étude du traitement et de la rééducation des séquelles d'hémiplégie. Paris

Ganne J M 1976 Interferential therapy. The Australian Journal of Physiotherapy 22 (3): 101–110

Ganne J M, Speculand B, Mayne L H, Goss A N 1979 Interferential therapy to promote union of mandibular fractures. Australian and New Zealand Journal of Surgery 49 (1): 81–83

Glick E N, Helal B 1976 Post-traumatic neurodystrophy. Hand 8 (1): 45–47

Gremieux G 1975 Traitement des algodystrophies. Révue Médicale 16 (27): 1786–1792

Gutmann E 1958 Die funktionelle Regeneration der peripheren Nerven. Akademie-Verlag, Berlin

Güttler P, Kleiditzsch J 1979 Die Anregung der Kallusbildung durch Interferenzströme. Deutsches Gesundheitswesen 34 (2): 91–94

Haag W 1979 Praktische Erfahrungen mit der Interferenzstromtherapie in der Gynäkologie. Der Frauenarzt 20 (1): 44–48

Hansjurgens A 1974 Dynamische Interferenzstromtherapie. Physikalische Medizin und Rehabilitation 15 (1): 24–28

Hansjurgens A 1978 Niederfrequente Reizströme. Medizinal Markt. Acta Medicotechnica 26 (3): 87–91

Harff J 1957 Vegetative Entgleisung (Sudecksche Dystrophie). Handbuch der Orthopädie 295: 763–782

Hauswirt O, Kracmar F 1959 Untersuchungen zur Interferenzstromtherapie. Archiv für Physikalische Therapie 12 (2): 138–139

Herzog M, Wilchelm K 1973 Der heutige Stand der operativen Versorgung peripherer Nervenverletzungen. Therapie der Gegenwart 112 (8): 1246

Hirthe D et al 1972 Einige Bemerkungen zur angeborenen Tibiapseudarthrose aus biochemischer Sicht. Beiträge zur Orthopädie und Traumatologie 19 (2): 82–86

Joutard H, de Bisschop G 1957 Electrogymnastique interférentielle statique et cinetique. Congrès de Médecine Physique de Marseille XII

Jung A, Gierlich K 1968 Die kombinierte Anwendung von

Ultraschall und Reizströmen. Physikalische Medizin und Rehabilitation 9 (9): 257–259

Kaindl F, Pärtan J 1953a Eine neue Kombinationsbehandlung bei arteriellen Durchblutungsstörungen. Wiener Zeitschrift für innere Medizin und ihre Grenzgebiete 7/8: 292–301

Kaindl F, Pärtan J, Warum F 1953b Behandlung der peripheren Kreislaufstörungen. Wiener Zeitschrift für innere Medizin und ihre Grenzgebiete 12: 465

Kleiditzsch J 1982 Bone union in experimental animals under the influence of bipolar rectangular pulse series and interferential current. Kurortologija i fizioterapija 19 (3): 139–141 (Bulgarian)

Klouchek-Popova E et al 1981 Experimental phytochemical, pharmacological and cytomorphological studies of the regenerative effect of the fractions C_1 and C_5 isolated from Calendula officinalis. Savremenna medicina 32 (8): 395–399 (Bulgarian)

Kolupaev G, Ulyanov M 1966 Electrosleep, electroanesthesia and electronarcosis. Moscow 32 (Russian)

Laabs W A et al 1980 New technique to stimulate healing of fractures by means of dynamic interferential current (DIC). 8th International Congress of Physical Medicine and Rehabilitation, Stockholm 25–29 Aug: 441–442

Laabs W A et al 1982a Knochenheilung und dynamischer Interferenzstrom (DIC) — Erste vergleichende tierexperimentalle Studie an Schafen.-Teil I: Experimentelles Vorgehen und histologische Ergebnisse. Langenbecks Archiv und Deutsche Zeitschrift für Chirurgie 356: 219–229

Laabs W A et al 1982b Knochenheilung und dynamischer Interferenzstrom (DIC).-Teil II: Physikalische und chemische Ergebnisse. Langenbecks Archiv und Deutsche Zeitschrift für Chirurgie 356: 231–241

Leeb H 1955 Über erste Erfahrungen mit der Anwendung interferierend Wechselströme bei entzündlichen Erkrankungen des weiblichen Genitales. Wiener Medizinische Wochenschrift 105 (47): 972–975

Leuthäusel W, Rugendorff E W 1978 Practical experience with interference current in therapy of autonomic urogenital disorder in man. Therapiewoche 28: 9019–9221

Makley I T et al 1967 The effect of reduced barometric pressure on fracture healing in rats. Journal of Bone and Joint Surgery 49A(5): 903

McQuire W A 1975 Treatment of stress incontinence and urinary freguence by electrotherapy and exercises. Physiotherapy 305–307

Meyer J 1952 Les courants croisés de moyenne fréquence à composante interférentielle de basse fréquence (courant de Nemec) en dermatologie. Synthèse de Sémiologie et Thérapeutique 23: 3

Meyer J 1953 Les courants rythmés contre les algies (courants de Nemec). Synthèse de Sémiologie et Thérapeutique 24: 6

Melnikov B 1966 Electrosleep, electroanesthesia and electronarcosis. Moscow 25 (Russian)

Mezzana M 1975 Rééducation des lésions traumatiques des nerfs radial, médian et cubital. Révue Médicale 16 (23): 1583–1592

Mucha C et al 1984 Zur diefereńzierten Übungsbehandlung beim Sudeck-Syndrom der Hand. Krankengymnastik 36 (12): 767–776

Müller H 1966 Über Elektroschlaf und Elektrotranquillisation. Bonn

Mutschler H 1952 Das neuartige Elektresiergerät 'Nemectrodyn' in der Orthopädie und Unfallchirurgie. Monatschrift für Unfallheilkunde 55 (4): 115–123

Nemec H 1966 Vademecum der Interferenzstromtherapie. Bonn

Nikoloff L 1955 Nemectrothérapie dans le traitement des séquelles de poliomyélite. Congrès National de Gymnastique Médicale. Naples

Nikolova L 1964 Effectiveness of the new physiotherapeutic method — interferential current in Sudeck's atrophy. Ortopedia i Travmatologia 1 (4): 261–265 (Bulgarian)

Nikolova L 1965 Treatment of deforming arthrosis with interferential current. Kurortologii i fizioterapija 2 (3): 111–114 (Bulgarian)

Nikolova L 1966a Die wirkung des Interferenzstromes bei Fazialis-nëuritis. Ärztliche Praxis 18 (13): 520–521

Nikolova L 1966b Efficience du courant interférentiel dans les cas périarthritis calcarea scapulo-humérale. Journal de Radiologie et d'Electrologie 47 (10): 521–524

Nikolova L 1966c The treatment of sports injuries with interferential current. ISRD, Proceedings of the Tenth World Congress. Wiesbaden, Germany September 11–17, 1966, p 161–162

Nikolova L 1967a Vergleichende Untersuchungen über therapeutische Erfolge der Interferenztherapie und anderer Methoden bei Arthrosis deformans. Physikalische Medizin und Rehabilitation 8 (3): 66–69

Nikolova L 1967b Interferenzstromtherapie bei Distorsionen, Kontusionen und Luxationen der Gelenke. Münchener Medizinische Wochenschrift 109 (11): 579–582

Nikolova L 1968a Oscillographic changes in Sudeck's dystrophy. Ortopedia i travmatologia 5 (4): 198–204 (Bulgarian)

Nikolova L 1968b Die modernen Elektrobehandlungsmethoden in der Therapie der Endarteritis obliterans. Therapie der Gegenwart 107 (2): 190–198

Nikolova L 1968c Das bewegungsgestörte Gelenk.- Rehabilitation der Bewegung. Ärztliche Praxis 20 (36): 1700–1705

Nikolova L 1968d Nouvelles possibilités de physiothérapie dans les cas d'endartérite oblitérante. Archives de l'Union médicale Balkanique 6 (6): 930

Nikolova L 1968e Notre expérience dans la rééducation du traumatisme sportif. Congrès International de Rééducation fonctionnelle, Nice 25–28 January 1968, p 324–326

Nikolova L 1969a Rehabilitation durch Interferenzstrom und Krankengymnastik bei Ellenbogengelankkontrakturen. Elektromedizin 14 (5): 202–205

Nikolova L 1969b Präventiv- und Nachbehandlung von Knochenbruchen. Therapiewoche 19 (43): 2128–2130

Nikolova L 1969c Physiotherapie und Thalassotherapie bei den Osteochondropathien. XIV Congrès International de Thalassothérapie, Roumanie Eforie Nord 27–31 May 1969, p 397–401

Nikolova L 1969d Influence of interferential current on bone tissue regeneration. Kurortologija i fizioterapija 6 (2): 70–75 (Bulgarian)

Nikolova L 1969e Special physiotherapy. Medicina i fizkultura Publishing House, 1st edn. Sofia, p 358–362 (Bulgarian)

Nikolova L 1969f Physiotherapeutische Rehabilitation bei Knochenbruchkomplikationen. Münchener Medizinische Wochenschrift 111 (11): 592–599

Nikolova L 1970a Personal experience of treatment of fractures and some of their complications. Voprossi kurortologii, fisioterapii i lechebnoi fisicheskoi kulturi 2: 157–160 (Russian)

Nikolova L 1970b New rehabilitation complexes of exercises in traumatic dislocations of the big joints. Kurortologija i fizioterapija 7 (3): 107–111 (Bulgarian)

Nikolova L 1970c Postoperative rehabilitation of meniscus lesions. Kurortologija i fizioterapija 7 (4): 158–162 (Bulgarian)

Nikolova L 1970d Niederfrequenztherapie mit Interferenzstrom bei Periarthritis humeroscapularis. Münchener Medizinische Wochenschrift 112 (11): 472–476

Nikolova L 1970e Physiotherapie der chirurgischen Erkrankungen. Urban und Schwarzenberg-Verlag, München

Nikolova L 1971a Treatment with interferential current. Medicina i fizkultura Publishing House. Sofia (Bulgarian)

Nikolova L 1971b Physikalische Therapie beim varikösen Symptomenkomplex. Therapie der Gegenwart 110 (5): 752–756

Nikolova L 1971c Die Rehabilitation durch Interferenzstrom bei Knochenbruchkomplikationen. Zeitschrift für physikalische Medizin 2 (4): 252–260

Nikolova L 1971d Le rôle de l'électrothérapie et de la kinésithérapie dans les cas de traumatisme de l'articulation du coude. Europa medicophysica 7 (3): 151–155

Nikolova L 1972a Die Bedeutung der Elektrotherapie bei der Rehabilitation von Patienten mit Speichenbruch loco typico. 6th Congreso Internacional de Medicina Fisica 2–6 July 1972 Barcelona, 2: 720–723

Nikolova L 1972b Rehabilitation bei traumatischer armneuritis durch Interferenzstrom. 6th Congreso Internacional de Medicina Fisica 2–6 July 1972 Barcelona, 2: 313–316

Nikolova L 1973a Remote results of electrotherapy in deforming arthrosis of knee joint. 1st National Congress of Physiotherapy, Health Resorts and Rehabilitation, Varna 17–20 October 1972. Medicina i fizkultura Publishing House Sofia, p 118–191 (Bulgarian)

Nikolova L 1973b Interferentne struje kod rehabilitacije neurita. Narodno zdravlje 29 (2–3): 46–51 (Serbian)

Nikolova L 1979 Treatment with interferential current. Medicina i fizkultura Publishing House. Sofia (Bulgarian)

Nikolova L 1983 Special physiotherapy. Medicina i fizkultura Publishing House, 3rd edn. Sofia, p 329, 402 (Russian)

Nikolova L 1984 Comparative studies on the influence of interferential current and microwaves in women with adnexial and tubal sterility. Akuserstvo i Ginekologija 23 (2): 158–161

Nikolova L, Balchev G 1969 Possibilities of physiotherapy in unfavourable intraarticular fractures of capitulum radii. Ortopedia i travmatologia 6 (4): 190–197 (Bulgarian)

Nikolova L, Balchev G 1972 Causes to which failure of the rehabilitation of traumatic intra- and periarticular lesions of the elbow is attributed. Ortopedia i travmatologia 9 (2): 93–100 (Bulgarian)

Nikolova L, Balchev G 1972 The effect of interferential current on the X-ray picture of Sudeck osteoporosis. Kurortologija i fizioterapija 9 (3): 122–127

Nikolova L, Balchev G 1977 Röntgenologischer Verlauf der Sudeck-Osteoporosis nach Interferenzstrombehandlung. Medizinische Klinik 72 (17): 751–753

Nikolova L, Davidov M 1978 Influence of interferential current on enzyme activity of traumatized nerve (Experimental study). Voprossi kurortologii, fisioterapii i lechebnoi fisicheskoi kulturi 6: 54–57 (Russian)

Nikolova L, Davidov M 1979 Anpassungsphänomene des Muskelgewebes bei traumatischer Neuritis nach Elektrotherapie. Zeitschrift für Physiotherapie 31 (4): 253–256

Nikolova L, Gerchev A 1972 Isolated traumatic injury of the tibiofibular syndesmosis and physiotherapeutic treatment of its residual effects. Ortopedia i travmatologia IX (3): 190–194 (Bulgarian)

Nikolova L, Ignatov N 1969 Physical therapy in small bone fragments. Ortopedia i travmatologia 6 (2): 76–80 (Bulgarian)

Nikolova L, Ivanov K 1974 Changes in skin temperature, oscillography and capillaroscopy under the effect of interferential current, ultrasound and microwaves. Kurortologija i fizioterapija 11 (2): 79–85 (Bulgarian)

Nikolova L, Ramadanov I 1977 Results from the treatment of tubal sterility with interferential current and microwaves. Akuserstvo i Ginecologija 16 (4): 257–262 (Bulgarian)

Nikolova L, Ratcheva T 1970 Thérapie, physioorophylaxie et résultats fonctionnels dans les fractures des os. Archives de l'Union Médicale Balkanique 8 (5–6): 621

Nikolova L, Takeva T 1980 Cytoenzymatic and ultrastructural characteristics of the condition of ovaries under the influence of centimetry waves. Voprossi kurortologii, fisioterapii i lechebnoi fisicheskoi kulturi 1: 31–35 (Russian)

Nikolova L et al 1980 Effect of interferent currents on experimental toxic hepatitis. Kurortologija i fizioterapija 17 (3): 105–110 (Bulgarian)

Nikolova L et al 1982 Hepatoprotective action of interferent current in experimentally induced d-galactosamine hepatitis — ultrastructural studies. Kurortologija i fizioterapija 19 (1): 5–12 (Bulgarian)

Nikolova L et al 1983 Magnetotherapy induced enhancement of regeneration of epithelization. Kurortologija i fizioterapija 20 (3): 100–110 (Bulgarian)

Nikolova L et al 1984a Comparative studies on stimulation of regeneration with interferential current. Kurortologija i fizioterapija 21 (2): 65–69 (Bulgarian)

Nikolova L et al 1984b Wirkungsmechanismus des Interferenzstromes und niederfrequenten Magnetfeldes bei der experimentellen Hepatitis (histologische und ultrastructurelle studien). Zeitschrift für Physiotherapie 36 (5): 311–316

Nikolova L et al 1984c D-Galactosamine-induced hepatitis: morphological and enzyme biochemical changes produced by interferential currents and low-frequency magnetic field. Physiotherapy 70 (8): 301–305

Nikolova L et al 1984d Influence of the interferential current and low-frequency magnetic field on the tissue-regeneration. Voprossi kurortologii, fisioterapii i lechebnoi fisicheskoi kulturi 3: 19–22

Nippel F J 1979 Interferential therapy. An advanced method in the management of pain. Annual Conference of the American Physics Therapy Association, 9 June 1979 Atlanta

Paleirah R, Cazejust J, Deville R 1956 Premiers résultats thérapeutiques par l'application des courants de moyenne fréquence interférentielle (courant de Nemec). Journal de Radiologie et d'Electrologie 37 (7/8): 606

Pärtan J, Schmid J, Warum F 1953 Über die Behandlung

entzündlicher und degenerativer Gelenkerkrankungen mit interferierenden Wechselströmen mittlerer Frequenzen. Wiener klinische Wochenschrift 65 (31): 624–628

Paunova M 1972 Treatment of enuresis nocturna and stress incontinence with interferential current. Voprossi kurortologii, fisioterapii i lechebnoi fisicheskoi kulturi 4: 354–357 (Russian)

Polster H 1965 Der gegenwärtige Stand der Interferenzstromtherapie in der Bundesrepublik Deutschland. Therapiewoche 4: 179–181

Portias L H 1977 Les algo-neurodystrophies réflexes des membres inférieurs. Semaine des Hôpitaux de Paris 53 (2): 133–138

Putan T 1966 Electrosleep, electroanesthesia and electronarcosis. Moscow (Russian)

Sachkov V 1966 Electrosleep, electroanesthesia and electronarcosis. Moscow (Russian)

Saitsev R S 1976 Treatment of injuries to nerve stems of the extremities. Medicina Leningrad (Russian)

Scheibe G 1960 Trophoneurotische Veränderungen bei der Sudeckschen Krankheit. Acta Neurovegetativa 21 (1–3): 141

Schlosser D 1973 Sudecksche Dystrophie nach Verletzungen des distalen Radiusendes und der Handwurzel. Langenbecks Archiv und Deutsche Zeitschrift für Chirurgie 334: 201–209

Speranskij A P, Svyanteko E S 1964 Influence of ultrasound on regeneration processes of the nervous system in injury to the peripheral nerve. Voprossi kurortologii, fisioterapii i lechebnoi fisicheskoi kulturi 72: 35–44

Steinbach M 1961 Die Behandlung mit Bernardischen Strömen. Kritische Überprüfung eines elektrotherapeutischen Verfahrens. Elektromedizin 6 (1): 7

Strougatskij V M, Kononova E 1968 Modern methods of examination and therapy in obstetrics and gynecology. Moscow, p 182–183 (Russian)

Terrier M 1954 Transformation d'une radiouermite par le nemectron. Bulletin de la Société Française de Dermatologie et de Syphiligraphie 61: 242

Thailhades C, de Bisschop G 1955 A propos du traitement des Algies viscérales par les courants d'interférence. Le Génie Médical V

Thorban W 1962 Posttraumatische Sudecksche Gliedmassendystrophie. Acta Neurovegetativa 25 (1): 1–62

Trueta G 1962 A theory of bone formation. Acta orthopaedica scandinavica 33 (3–4): 190–198

Wagner W 1960 Das Sudeck-Syndrom. Maudrich Verlag, Wien

Willengger H 1971 Knochenregeneration und Transplantation. Primäre und sekundäre Knochenbruchheilung. Der Chirurg 42 (6): 241

Woeber K, Polster H G 1966 Über den derzeitigen Stand der interferenzstrom- und Farben- Bzw- Farblichttherapie. Excerpta Medica — International Congress Series 107: 471–475

Wolf S 1956 Interferenzstrom-Therapie. Elektromedizin 1 (3): 77

Index